Haircutting Basics

An easy, step-by-step guide to cutting hair the professional way

Martha G. Fernandez

Illustrated by

Dacil Hernandez

GOOD LIFE PRODUCTS, INC.
P.O. BOX 5122
HIALEAH, FL 33014-1122

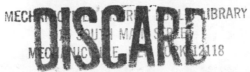

Haircutting Basics

*An easy step-by-step guide to
cutting hair the professional way*

Martha G. Fernandez

illustrated by:

Dacil Hernandez

Published by:

*Good Life Products, Inc.
Post Office Box 5122
Hialeah, FL 33014-1122 U.S.A.*

Library of Congress Cataloging-in-Publication Data.

Fernandez, Martha G.,   1954-
    Haircutting basics :   an easy, step-by-step guide to cutting hair
the professional way / Martha G. Fernandez : illustrated by Dacil Hernandez

    p.   cm.
    Bibliography: p.
    Includes index
    ISBN 0-944460-11-9   ISBN 0-944460-12-7 (pbk.)
    1. Haircutting.   I. Title.
TT970. F47 1988
646.7' 242--dc19   87-28945
                                                CIP

DISCLAIMER

Anyone who wishes to cut hair with accuracy must expect to dedicate time to practice and gain expertise.

The purpose of this book is to inform, educate and entertain its readers. The author and Good Life Products, Inc. shall have neither liability nor responsibility to any person or entity with respect to any loss or damage caused or alleged to be caused directly or indirectly by the information contained in this book.

ATTENTION SCHOOLS

THIS BOOK IS AVAILABLE AT SPECIAL QUANTITY DISCOUNT

FOR DETAILS WRITE TO:

GOOD LIFE PRODUCTS, INC.
SPECIAL SALES DEPT.
DIANA JOHNSTONE
P.O. BOX 5122
HIALEAH, FL 33014-1122

TABLE OF CONTENTS

CHAPTER II--Technique

CHAPTER III--More technique 151

How to cut wisps of hair
How to layer bangs
How to spike the hair of the top
How to cut the top for forward motion
How to cut the top for backward motion
How to cut ducktails
How to blow-style the hair

CHAPTER 1V--Analizing the hair 161

Hair elasticity
Shampooing and conditioning the hair
Brushing the hair

APPENDIX

ACKNOWLEDGMENTS

Writing a book is like having a baby. It has to be created, be nurtured and be launched. It also takes the labor of many people. I am grateful to all.

I am grateful to my friend and editor Maria V. Vila, for her valuable revision and critique of this edition.

I am grateful to my husband Gilbert, for his cooperation, involvement, encouragement and support. The enthusiam that he provided made this book a reality.

I am grateful to several friends, professionals and teachers who in many different ways helped me create this book.

Finally, I am grateful to Director Diana Jonhstone for having the patience, optimism and commitment that this project required.

INTRODUCTION

Haircutting is the art of changing the hair into a style, mainly with the purpose of creating a more attractive and neater appearance. The art of cutting hair has been practiced from prehistoric times among all kinds of cultures. In ancient times hairdressing demanded processing and adornment of the hair. Today there is a definite choice for wash-and-wear haircuts, that can be styled in a conservative or sophisticated fashion to reflect the individual's character.

There are many ways to cut hair, and today's students are in need of material that explains and shows the how-to of cutting hair. This book was designed for beginners who are in the process of training to become future haircutters; for the graduates of beauty school who haven't developed a haircutting technique of their own, and for persons who have interest in learning an easy haircutting technique to take care of their friends' and families' hairstyling needs.

One of the first tasks in this book was to keep technical terminology to a minimum, and to choose a format in which to present this material. I have organized the material from basic and essential information to complex training, needed for the development of the skills. I have also introduced some advanced instruction to prepare the individual for more progress.

Related material has been compiled in Sections to be used for quick reference. For those who have the basic notions, I have prepared the haircutting Sections so they can directly start with the technique and skip the fundamental and informational portions.

Many people are afraid to cut hair because they think that cutting is complicated. Haircutting is a skill that requires practice just as typewriting or playing the guitar. Once the beginner has learned and practiced this method, it will not be forgotten; it will provide the foundation to learn advanced methods to create different effects in the hair.

This book presents a standard technique that is simple, effective and easy to learn. Repetition of the haircutting steps aids learning by helping memorize the technique and develop speed and accuracy. A Glossary, Index and illustrations have been included to make this book completely clear to any audience, young or old, native or foreign, amateur or beauty student.

With this idea in mind, this book has a unique method of providing the instruction needed to cut hair with precision. Later, through practice of this technique, the individual will develop the experience necessary to become a great haircutter.

This book should first be read thoroughly for an overview of the subject. The second reading should be done with a friend on whom to practice the cutting technique. To practice the technique choose a haircut, place the book on a table and follow the steps indicated. The type is large enough to be read at a distance.

Here, then, is an easy haircutting technique that this author believes anyone can understand and learn.

Chapter I

FUNDAMENTALS

There are many variables to a good haircut--the tools, the type and condition of the hair, the technique employed, and the facial characteristics and physique of the individual. To obtain successful haircuts you need to have knowledge of these variables; they're the fundament to understand why the hair behaves as it does and what results will be obtained when you give a haircut.

In this Chapter you will learn about those variables to prepare you for Chapter II--haircutting technique in depth.

A. TOOLS

The Scissors

There are a wide range of haircutting scissors in the market. Once you have spent some time cutting hair with different types of scissors, you'll be able to determine which one suits you best. In precision haircutting the hair is cut with the tips of the scissors, that's why I recommend to use the mini-scissors. Since they are small (from four to five and a half inches), they fit the hand comfortably and the short blades give you better control when cutting sides and corners. *Fig. 1.1.*

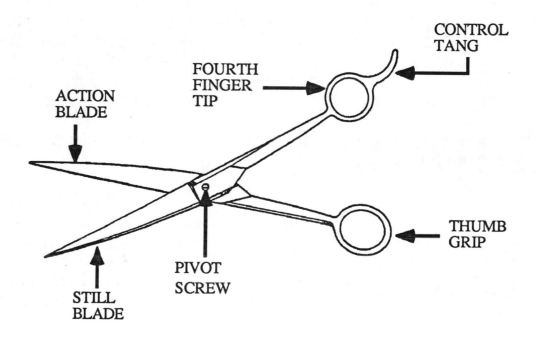

Fig 1.1

Usually long bladed scissors are used in barber styling techniques in combination with the comb where the lengths to cut are long across the head. To cut the layers with uniformity using this technique, long bladed scissors are necessary. Small scissors would cut small sections and the layers would be uneven.

The scissors' control tang is not necessary, but try it, it may help you maintain the scissors in balance while you cut.

Prices for scissors range from a few dollars to over a hundred. You'll have to determine which one is affordable to you. It is not necessary to invest in an expensive pair of scissors, but those with low quality will cut unevenly. There are a wide selection of scissors made in Solingen, West Germany. Solingen is a city famous for its steel and iron ware. The scissors made there are exported to all parts of the world The ice-tempered stainless are good and reasonably priced. Check the Appendix of this book for some distributors' adresses, to obtain information about where to buy good quality scissors.

The blades should be dried after each haircut. Residues of hair should be cleaned. The pivot screw and the inside of the blades should be kept clean and oiled with clipper type oil. When needed, the blades of your fine shears should be sharpened by an experienced sharpening and honing expert. They know what the needs of different types of scissors are, for optimum sharpness and edge holding durability. I have had scissors ruined by grinders that have completely removed the teeth or broken the blades. So be smarted than I was; ask for a guaranteed job.

Be careful with your scissors. If you drop them the points may be damaged and they may lose their pivot screw adjustment.

The pivot screw should not be tight or loose. To find out if it is properly adjusted, hold the scissors horizontally by the thumb grip (pivot screw facing you); open wide the upper grip and let it drop. If the tips of the scissors are more than one-eight of an inch open, the screw is tight; if the tips are closed, the screw is loose. The tips of the scissors should stop at a distance of one-eight of an inch from each other when the still blade drops. Proper adjustment will prevent damage to the hair and to the scissors. *Fig. 1.2.*

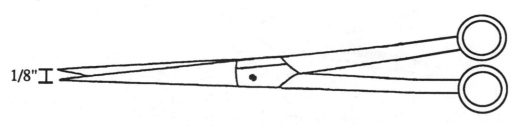

PROPERLY ADJUSTED SCISSORS

Fig. 1.2

Thinning Shears

Thinning shears are used to reduce hair bulk. There are two types of thinning shears.

a) <u>Notched Single Edge Scissor</u> *Fig. 1.3*.

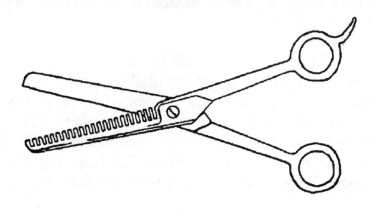

Fig. 1.3

b) <u>Notched Double Edge Scissor</u>

Shears with teeth on one blade take off more hair than those with teeth on both blades. *Fig. 1.4*.

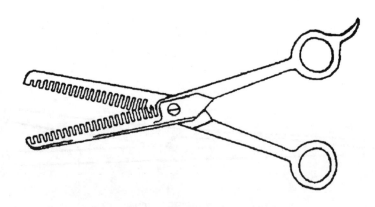

Fig. 1.4

These are some general rules to thin out the hair correctly with thinning shears:

1) Thinning is done in the underlying layers of the hair; the top layers should be longer to cover the hair that has been thinned out.

2) Don't thin out too much hair.

3) Don't thin hairline hair.

4) Don't thin the hair too close to the scalp. Start thinning the hair at least one inch away from the scalp.

5) Thin the hair in small even sections.

6) Place the scissors in a vertical or a diagonal direction to avoid steps in the hair. Straight hair will show a chopped look.

7) Work your way from the top to the bottom in spaced intervals.

8) Don't close the scissors partially. It will give more damage to the hair.

9) Don't thin the hair before a permanent wave. You need even sections of hair to roll it easily on the rods.

A precision haircut cannot be accomplished if it involves thinning the hair. The reason is that thinning gives the hair uneven lengths. To thin the hair correctly, the techniques must be practiced, otherwise you can spoil a good haircut. I prefer to use the thinning shears to create special effects, or to give volume to some areas of the hairstyle. You will learn some of these techniques in Chapter III.

Slithering is another method to thin the hair. The scissors are slid up and down the underside of a strand of hair; they are closed slightly on each stroke toward the head, then opened as they are brought back. This method can scratch and partially cut the cortex. The razor may also be used to thin out the hair. Razor cutting and thinning sharpens the ends, scratches and creates split and dry flyaway ends. Neither method is recommended.

Many people note that when their hair was thinned out it became unmanageable after a couple of weeks. The shorter ends, as they grew, pushed the longer hair making it seem even bulkier. People with coarse, curly and of thick density hair often want it thinned out. Usually this types of hair tend to push more as they grow. So, unless you plan to give an exotic style that requires thinning, it is best to shape the hair with a precision haircut--it will last longer and with the right haircut you can diminish bulk.

Electric Clippers

It is faster and safer to cut hair off the neck with the clippers than with the scissors or the razor. Also they are useful to trim and retouch the hairline, the sideburns, the moustache and beard. There are also techniques to give an entire haircut solely with clippers. However, the clippers used to cut facial hair are different to those used to cut scalp hair. The hair on a man's face is much thicker and coarser than the hair on the scalp, and a fine pair of clippers will get damaged if they are regularly used to cut facial hair. The blades of the clippers should be dried and the hair should be brushed off the blades with a small brush. Be gentle when using the clippers, if you push too hard on the skin you'll cause scratches and uncomfort. When clipping a man's neckline, make sure to follow its natural shape and avoid cutting above the hairline. On page thirty-three you will find more details about how to cut the hairline area. *Fig. 1.5*.

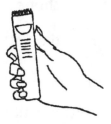

Fig. 1.5

The Comb

The hair will be handled better with a hard, sturdy comb. One half should have the teeth set wide apart; the other fine closed set teeth. The wide teeth are used to untangle hair. To untangle hair start at the ends and work your way up to the top, half an inch at a time. The fine teeth are used to smooth the hair once it has been untangled. Either side can be used to lift the hair. You may want to use the wide teeth to lift thick hair, and the closed set teeth to lift fine hair. *Fig. 1.6*. Combs that lose their teeth should be discarded, they cause damage and comb the hair unevenly.

BACK

WIDE TEETH   FINE THEETH

Fig. 1.6

B. THE HAIR

Hair Structure

Hair is mostly protein. When observed under a microscope you can see that the hair has three layers *(fig. 1.7)*. The cuticle is the outer layer composed of tiny overlapping scales made of hard protein. This hard protein is called keratin; it protects the hair and holds moisture.

The hair looks dull and dry when the cuticle is open or broken. Some of this damage occurs if the hair is over-processed with chemicals, burned by a hot drier applied too close to the hair, over-exposure to the sun or chlorine, and even by brushing it and pulling it when wet. Alkaline products applied to the hair will open the cuticle and make it sensitive to breakage.

pH balanced shampoos and conditioners are recommended to close the cuticle's scales and make the hair feel soft and look shiny.

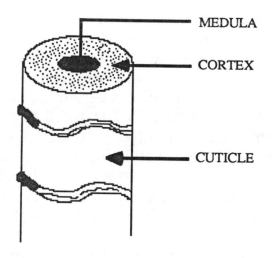

Fig. 1.7

The cortex is the layer next to the cuticle. This is where melanin, the pigment that gives the hair color, is produced. The medulla is the innermost layer of cells in the hair. The purpose of the medulla is not known. *Fig. 1.7.*

Form, Texture, and Density of Hair

Each hair grows out of a tiny tube in the scalp called the follicle. In its base the papilla produces the cells necessary for hair growth and it nourishes the follicle with blood and oxygen. If the papilla is damaged or destroyed, it will not produce hair. *Fig. 1.8.*

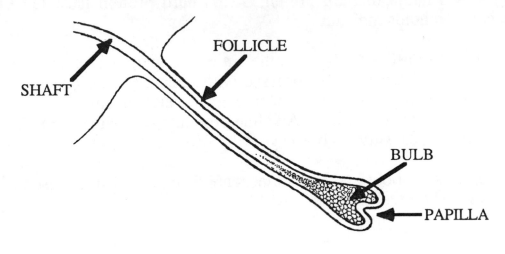

Fig. 1.8

There are four major forms of hair: 1) straight, 2) wavy, 3) curly, and 4) super-curly. The shape of the hair follicle determines the form that the hair will have. Detailed in figure 1.9 are the different relationships between the shape of the hair follicle and the forms of hair that will result. Each of these forms can be fine, medium or coarse in texture. The texture is determined by the size of the cortex that makes the hair shaft thicker or thinner. Fine textured hair is soft and shiny; it tends to go limp and flat and won't hold a set. Medium textured hair has body and bounce; it has a strong direction, so it's better to style it following its own natural pattern. The ends may feel coarse, dry and prone to split ends. With rich conditioners the hair may go limp. Coarse hair lacks shine, is dry, bulky and wiry; it requires extra care such as rich conditioners, the right cut, and styling aids to control its bulk.

Hair density refers to the amount of hairs per square inch. Blonds have the most density, brown and black haired follow, and red heads have the least density. Rather than dealing with the number of hairs per square inch we'll define density as thin, medium or thick. To determine the density of a specific head of hair look for these clues: Is the scalp visible when the hair is wet or dry? Do conditioners make the hair flat? Is the hair bushy? Does it need gel or other styling aids to control it? The density is thin if the scalp shows through the hair and conditioners flatten the hair. The density is medium if the scalp does not show when the hair is wet or dry and it does not appear bushy. The hair is thick if the hair has lots of bulk and styling aids are needed to control it.

Usually curly and super-curly hair (because they coil out from the scalp), as well as any hair that's coarse, tend to be bulky. Black hair is specially fragile because is has a thin cortex, and it is usually processed with strong harsh chemicals that make it dryer and prone to breakage. These types of hair will look more attractive with a layered cut to shape the hair, reduce its volume, and eliminate the split ends. However, fine hair, also with a thin cortex will appear thicker with a blunt cut. *Fig. 1.9.*

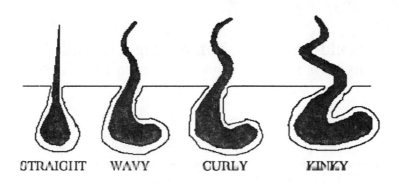

STRAIGHT   WAVY   CURLY   KINKY

Fig. 1.9

Shape of the Follicle	Forms of Hair
round	straight hair
oval	wavy hair
almost flat	curly hair
flat	super-curly hair

Growth of Hair

Hair length is the distance between the base of the hair to the end of the hair. *Fig. 1.10.*

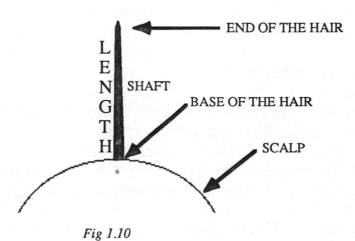

Fig 1.10

21

The hair shaft grows about half an inch per month. Short hair is closer to the scalp; it shows uneven length sooner than long hair. You can recommend monthly trims for short hair. Long hair can wait six to eight weeks to be trimmed.

Healthy unwet hair stretches up to one-fifth of its normal length when held tautly, springing back to its original length when released. Wet with water it will stretch almost half its length. Therefore, when you cut it wet and stretched it'll be shorter after it dries. *Fig. 1.11.*

Special care should be taken when cutting hair with body, coarse or curly. After the hair dries and curls it will be shorter than hair that is straight.

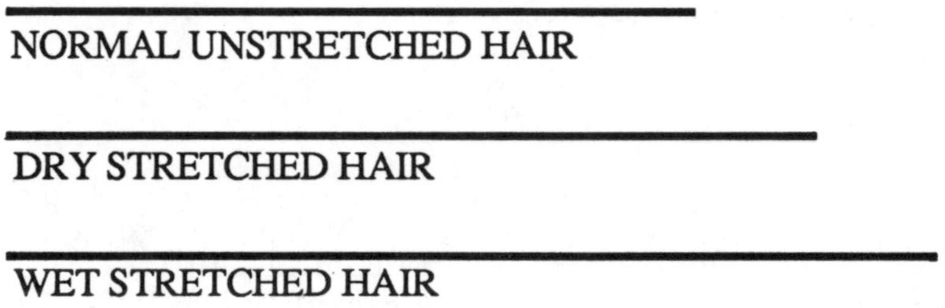

NORMAL UNSTRETCHED HAIR

DRY STRETCHED HAIR

WET STRETCHED HAIR

Fig. 1.11

All hair go through a process of three different phases called Anagen, Catagen and Telogen. The papilla controls these phases. Anagen is the growing phase; most of the hair is in this phase which lasts two to six years. After the Anagen, there is a resting period called Catagen during which the follicle is dormant. At the end of the cycle comes the Telogen phase. In this phase the hair falls each day in a shedding process, replacing the old hair with new. Age, failing health, trauma, pregnancy, drugs, poor diet, and constantly pulling the hair with pony tails may cause temporary baldness or slow hair growth.

Many people believe that shaving the children's hair will stimulate the growth of strong, abundant hair. Shaving will not change the kind of hair a person has. The genes determine the papilla and follicle located in the interior layers of the scalp and it will not change by shaving the hair shaft. • As the child grows the hair will go throrough several stages, it may become stronger and thicker, or remain fine.

C. EXERCISES

The following exercises have been designed to help you accomplish the objectives listed below. Practice them carefully to be able to learn the haircutting technique explained in this book. Once you become proficient in your practice of these exercises, you can move on to the next Section. If you have had some instruction and are familiar with these objectives, go on to more complex material.

Objectives:

1) To be able to name the parts of the hand.
2) To be able to hold the scissors correctly.
3) To be able to hold the scissors and the comb correctly.
4) To be able to hold the scissors and the comb correctly, while combing the hair.
5) To be able to hold and move the scissors, the comb and the hair correctly, while cutting the hair.

Parts of the hand

The dominant hand (meaning your right if you are right handed, or your left if you are left handed), manipulates the scissors and combs the hair. The opposite hand holds the hair to be cut, determines how much hair will be cut, and holds the comb while the dominant hand is cutting. The following terms will be used when referring to the hand. Familiarize yourself with these terms to be able to understand the explanation of the exercises that follow. *Fig.1.12.*

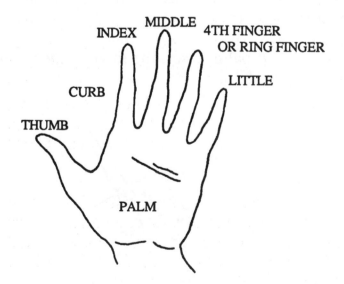
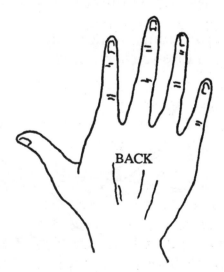

Fig. 1.12

Exercise #1. Hold the scissors with your dominant hand. Face the scissors' pivot screw toward your chest. Insert the thumb in the thumb grip and the ring finger in the fourth finger grip. If your scissors have control tang rest your little finger on it. Fingers should be inserted up to the first joint. Once you have the correct hand position, open and close the scissors only moving the action blade. Your thumb will be doing the work, while the still blade, controlled by the ring finger, remains motionless.

Action: Open, close. Repeat increasing speed. *Fig. 1.13.*

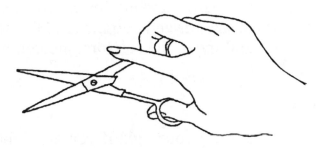

Fig. 1.13

Exercise #2. Hold the scissors as practiced. Close the blades; and keeping the ring finger inside the fourth finger grip, remove the thumb from its grip and hold the scissors in the palm of your hand. Now, insert the thumb back into its grip and open and close the scissors three times as learned in the previous exercise. Repeat the entire exercise twenty times trying to increase speed.

Action: Remove the thumb, hold scissors in palm, insert the thumb, open and close scissors. Repeat increasing speed. *Fig. 1.14.*

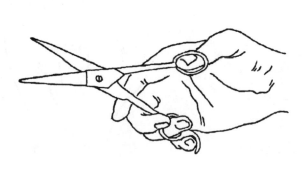

Fig. 1.14

Exercise #3. With scissors in the palm of your hand, take hold of the back of the comb with your index finger and thumb of the same hand. In this position, comb the hair of a friend or a wig lifting the hair up and letting it drop. Repeat ten times. Start on the left side of the head and move towards the right. (Beware of the tips of the scissors. In this position someone could be accidentally hurt).

Action: Hold closed scissors and comb the hair up, drop hair. Repeat increasing speed. *Fig. 1.15*.

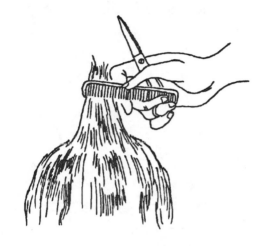

Fig 1.15

Exercise #4. With scissors and comb in the palm of your dominant hand, comb the hair up and hold it between the middle and index fingers of your opposite hand. Drop the hair, and repeat the procedure five times moving from left to right.

Action: Hold closed scissors and comb, comb hair up, hold hair with fingers, drop hair. Repeat. *Fig. 1.16*.

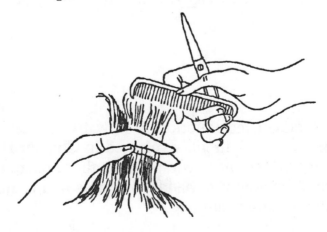

Fig. 1.16

25

Exercise #5. Repeat exercise four, but do not drop the hair. Instead, transfer the comb to the opposite hand and hold the teeth in the curb of your hand, using the thumb to secure it in place. Insert the thumb in the scissors' grip and pretend cutting. Remove the thumb from its grip and hold the scissors in the palm of your hand. Return the comb to the dominant hand. Drop the hair. Repeat the exercise combing the hair from left to right, transferring the comb back and forth, trying to gain speed.

Action: Hold comb and closed scissors with dominant hand (ring finger in its grip), comb hair up, hold hair with fingers, transfer comb, insert thumb in its grip, pretend cutting, hold closed scissors in palm, transfer comb back to dominant hand, and drop hair. Repeat. *Fig. 1.17.*

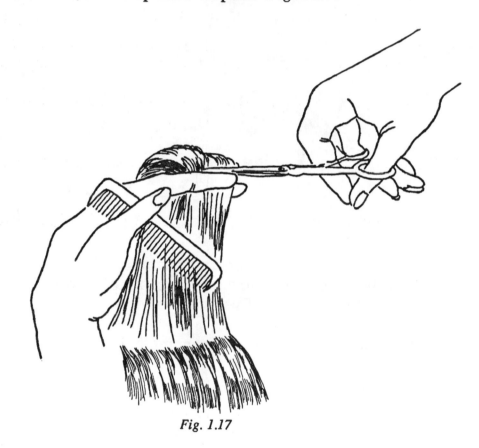

Fig. 1.17

Now you have had an introduction to how to handle the tools and the hair. Later while giving the practice haircuts explained in Chapter II, you will gain control and speed. Remember that the more you practice these exercises the better prepared you will be to cut hair. The goal is to handle the tools in an automatic way so you can fully concentrate on the cutting technique.

D. LEARN YOUR ANGLES

In the course of this book you will give several practice haircuts; some of the haircuts will be layered.

Layers are progressive graduations of the hair, from short to long, or from long to short. In order to cut layers, small sections of hair are elevated and cut. According to the elevation you give to the hair, you will accomplish a different length, and therefore, a different hairstyle. It is important that you learn how to measure elevations and know how to use them when cutting hair.

When you lift the hair from the scalp, you make an angle. An angle is measured in degrees. To cut hair you will form an angle with the surface of the scalp and the hair. The separation between the scalp and the hair will mark the degrees of the angle.

The following figures show the angles that you will use in the cutting technique explained in Chapter II. The small round symbol next to the numbers means degree.

Look at figure 1.18. The separation between these two lines is a ninety-degree angle.

Figure 1.19 shows a forty-five-degree angle which is one half of the ninety-degree angle.

A 180 degree angle is a straight line; two ninety-degree angles added together. See figure 1.20.

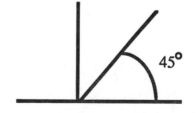

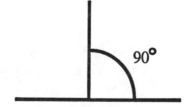

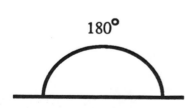

Fig 1.18   Fig. 1.19   Fig. 1.20

If you are told to elevate the hair at a ninety-degree angle there are two things you need to remember:

1. Think of an imaginary line, or place a ruler touching the head at the base of the hair you are holding. *Fig. 1.21*.

2. Elevate the hair at a ninety-degree angle from this line. If you have difficulty doing this, place your hand flat on the scalp with a strand of hair between your fingers. Lift your hand straight out from this point and you will have a ninety-degree angle.

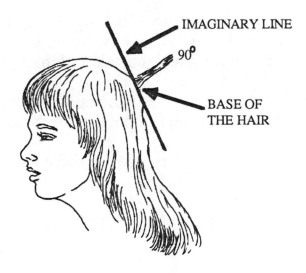

Fig. 1.21

Note that when you elevate the hair at a ninety-degree angle the hair seems to come straight out from the scalp following the roundness of the head. *Fig. 1.22*.

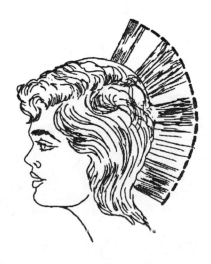

Fig. 1.22

Practice the same method elevating the hair at a forty-five-degree angle.   See *Fig. 1.23*.

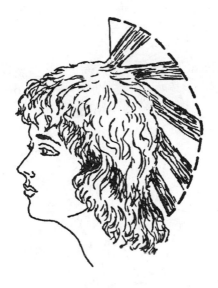

Fig. 1.23

If you are told to elevate the hair at a 180 degree angle, you will hold it straight up to coincide with the top half of the imaginary line as in figure 1.24.

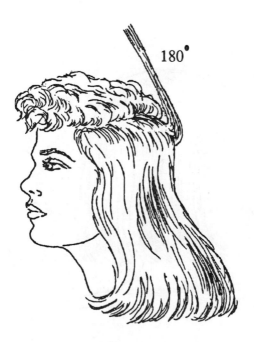

Fig. 1.24

29

If you look at figure 1.25, you can see a combination of all the angles discussed and how they relate to each other.

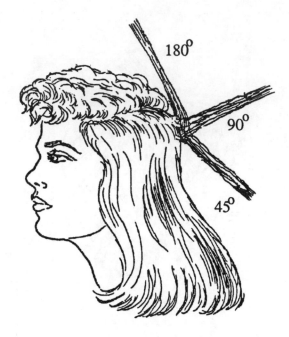

Fig. 1.25

Another term we need to mention is "zero elevation." When you are told to hold the hair at zero elevation, keep the hair close to the person's body, (occipital bone, neck or back). Hair that is cut at zero elevation has no layers. This hair is called "one-length." *Fig. 1.26.*

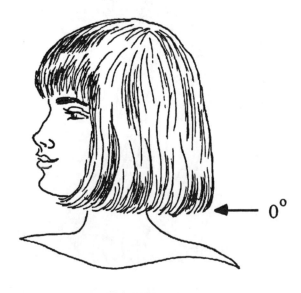

Fig. 1.26

E. PARTS OF THE HEAD

These terms indicate the parts of the head. They are mentioned in the Sections that follow. Please be familiar with them. *Fig. 1.27*.

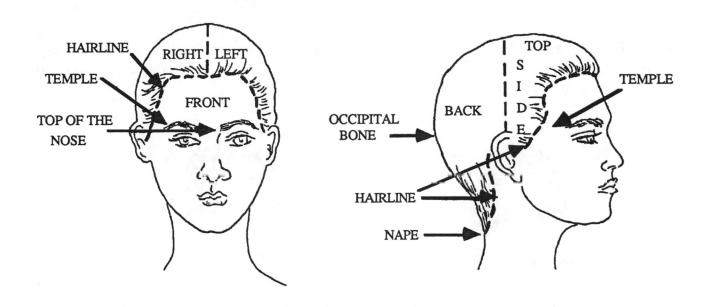

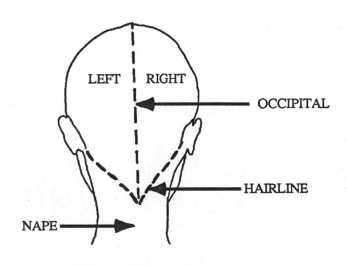

Fig. 1.27

F. A WORD ABOUT GUIDES

This section has the purpose of giving an overview of the guides you will be using in the cutting technique explained in Chapter II. Be familiar with these definitions. As the study progresses, you'll be able to relate this information to the actual cutting technique. Refer to this Section whenever you have questions about the guides.

Guides are points of reference to help you determine the length of each layer being cut. In symmetrical cuts *see fig 1.28,* guides will also help you determine if the lengths are equally long on either side of the head.

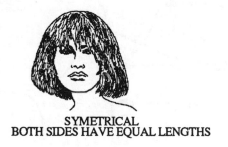

SYMETRICAL
BOTH SIDES HAVE EQUAL LENGTHS

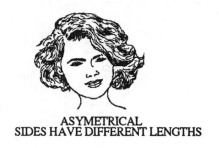

ASYMETRICAL
SIDES HAVE DIFFERENT LENGTHS

Fig. 1.28

The technique explained in Chapter II employs the following guides:

Outline or perimeter: The perimeter is the edge of the haircut. *Fig. 1.29.* It sets the length and shape that the hair is to have around the face and the back.

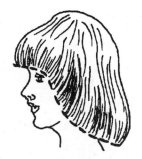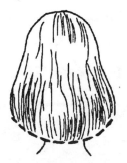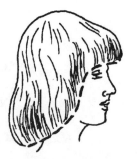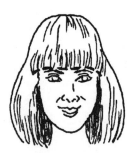

THE BROKEN LINE INDICATES THE PERIMETER.

Fig. 1.29

Once the perimeter's length and shape have been defined, it can be elevated at a forty-five-degree or a ninety-degree angle to serve as an initial guide to length of the hair above it. In this way you will give layers to the hair. *Fig. 1.30.*

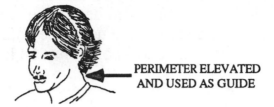

PERIMETER ELEVATED
AND USED AS GUIDE

Fig. 1.30

Hairline: When cutting the outline you will want to leave a distance from the hairline to the perimeter. Never cut above the hairline unless you are giving an exotic haircut. For a very short haircut you can cut at hairline level in the back and the sides. However, in the front you'll have to be careful. If you cut too close to the hairline the cut will look odd, or the hair may stick up. *Fig. 1.31.*

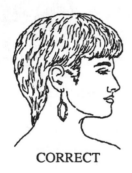 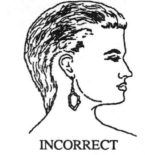

CORRECT   INCORRECT

Fig 1.31

Checkpoints: The purpose of the checkpoint is to indicate the right length to give to the layers before you start cutting sections. It will save you having to retrace your steps and cut more if you left the hair too long, or the possibility of cutting the hair too short, an irreversible mistake.

For example, some types of hair such as straight coarse oriental hair need to have enough length to make the hair heavier--the weight will keep it from sticking up. Other types such as thinning hair need to be cut short enough to produce the volume and bounce it needs or it will lay flat making the scalp visible.

There are two checkpoints: crown-level checkpoint and top-level checkpoint.

Crown-level checkpoint is a one-quarter inch strand of hair located in the center of the crown. Sometimes in the midst of a cowlick or cowlicks. It serves as a guide to determine the length of top, side and back layers. You will use it in all layered haircuts such as the one-level, bi-level with long-layered back, and long-layered styles.

To make this checkpoint, cut the ends of one-quarter inch strand of crown hair and drop it *see fig. 1.32*. When this hair curls the ends must touch the back of the head. If it is cut too short it will stick up; if too long, it will lay flat. You can easily determine the right length by cutting the ends a bit at a time and dropping the hair to see how it curls. If you still have problems to determine where to cut the crown-level checkpoint, place your comb flat on top of the head; the point where the head separates from the comb will indicate where the checkpoint must be located. *Fig. 1.33*.

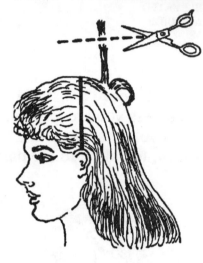

Fig. 1.32

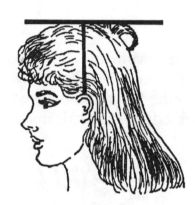

Fig. 1.33

Top-level checkpoint is a one-quarter inch strand of hair located on the top, at joining point of ear-to-ear parting. It will be your guide to determine the length of top and side layers.

This checkpoint is used in haircuts that will be layered in the top only, or in the top and sides with one-length in the back. Haircuts such as bi-level with bobbed back, bob variation, and bob with one-level top will have the top-level checkpoint. If you give this checkpoint the right length, the hair will curl and bounce touching the crown of the head. *Fig. 1.34*.

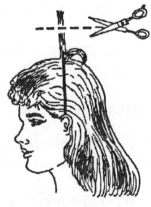

Fig. 1.34

Shoulders: Help to indicate the back lengths. Above the shoulders is a good length for a bob. *Fig. 1.35*.

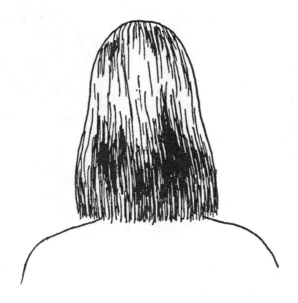

Fig. 1.35

Eyebrows: Help determine the front length. According to the style desired you will cut above the eyebrows, eyebrow level or below the eyebrows. *Fig. 1.36*.

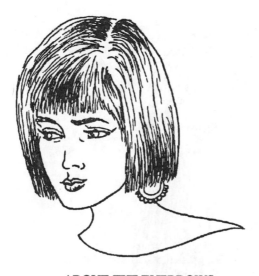 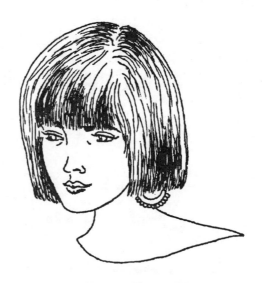

ABOVE THE EYEBROWS   UNDER THE EYEBROWS

Fig. 1.36

Mouth, jaw or chin: Serve to indicate top or side lengths. *Fig. 1.37.*

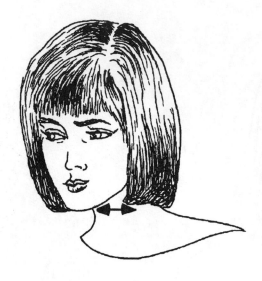 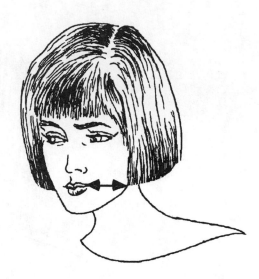

Fig. 1.37

Temples: When the hair is very short in the front and sides, they serve as joining point of front and side outline. To give more length to the hair, cut it below the temples. Also the temples serve as a guide to make the triangle parting on the top. *Fig. 1.38.*

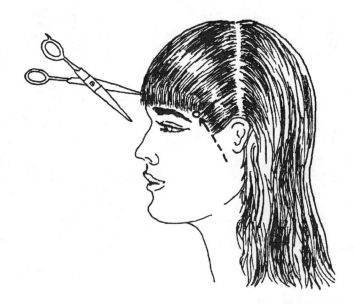

Fig. 1.38

Ears: Serve as a guide to length on both sides of the face. Example: above the ears, mid-ear, and below the ears are common lengths for the side hair. *Fig. 1.39.*

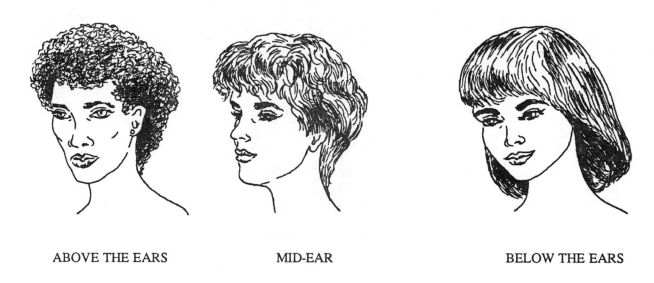

ABOVE THE EARS   MID-EAR   BELOW THE EARS

Fig. 1.39

Nose: Helps you center the top layer and determine the front length. Example: the top, the bridge and the tip of the nose are common lengths for the front hair. *Fig. 1.40.*

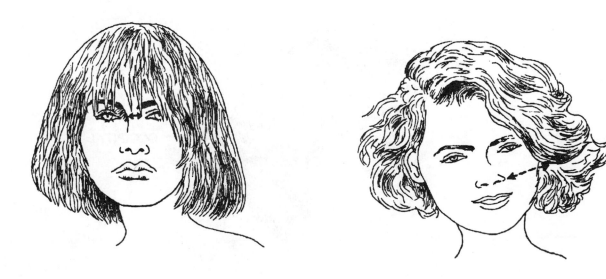

Fig. 1.40

Top layer: Serves as guide to the length of side and back layers. *Fig. 1.41.*

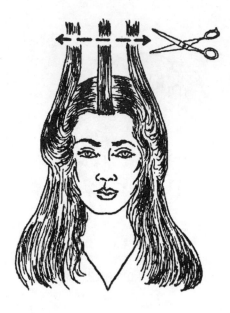

Fig. 1.41

Occipital bone: Serves as a guide to indicate where to stop layering a wedge haircut. It also serves to indicate the back partings of a bob haircut. *Fig. 1.42.*

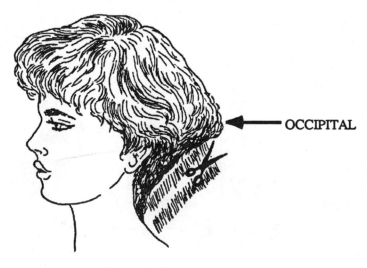

OCCIPITAL

Fig. 1.42

Sections and layers: Sections are divisions within the partings. *Fig. 1.43.*. They are approximately one to two inches wide. Some beginners feel that smaller sections are easier to cut, others say that larger sections help them follow the guide better. With smaller sections more precision will be accomplished. When you elevate the section at a chosen degree and cut it, each hair will have a different length. Each length is a layer, *see fig. 1.44.*. Sections can be cut in any direction and at any degree according to the desired effect of the final cut. To make clean sections, comb the hair down, part the section, and comb the hair at either side in a horizontal direction. *Fig. 1.44.*

Starting from the second consecutive section, include one-quarter inch of hair from the previous completed section. This quarter inch will not be cut again; it will be a guide to length to your new section. With this procedure you'll be overlapping and blending the sections, and you won't miss any hair. *Fig. 1.43.*

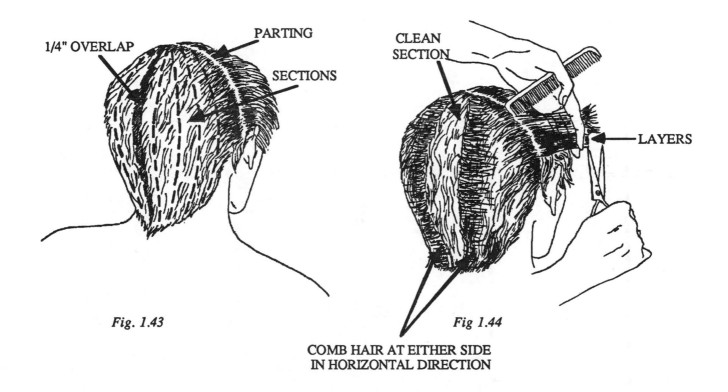

Fig. 1.43

Fig 1.44

COMB HAIR AT EITHER SIDE
IN HORIZONTAL DIRECTION

On page thirty we spoke about zero elevation. A sequence of horizontal sections are made to cut the hair at zero elevation; this way it is easier to follow the guide to the length. The technique to cut horizontal sections of hair will be detailed in

G. LEARN YOUR INCHES

A person's perception of one inch could range from one-quarter inch to three inches. To understand as clearly as possible what the person wants, you will show him with your fingers how much hair you are planning to cut, making sure this is what he wants.

Exercise

Place your thumb and index fingers at each end of the different lines on the figure below. Lift your hand trying to keep the separation between the fingers and observe. Now start all over again, this time without looking at the lengths try to duplicate them. Then match the separation of your fingers to the length chosen. Repeat until you can perfectly match the lengths. *Fig. 1.45.*

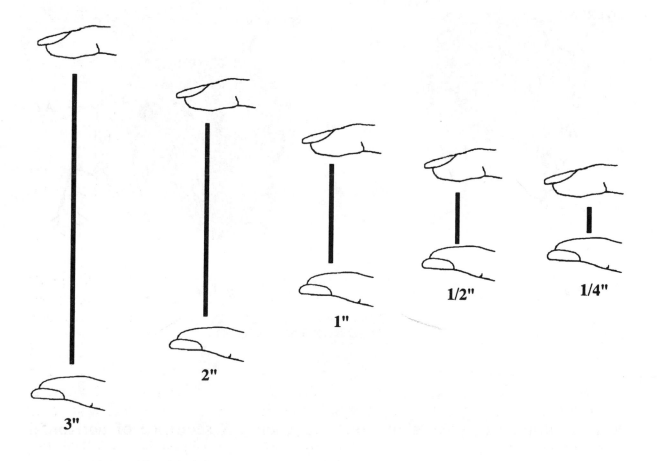

Fig. 1.45

H. CORRECTIVE HAIRCUTTING

Most people want a haircut that harmonizes with their personality and life-style, but it may not suit their type of hair. For example, they may have a picture of a haircut that requires thick hair with body, but their hair is limp; or they may show you a cut for straight hair, but they have super-curly hair. This is when you should explain the limitations that their type of hair imposes. They need to accept what Nature has given them and work with it to find an acceptable look that will enhance their good features.

The first step is to match the haircut to the form, texture and density of the hair. You will have to find out if they are willing to dedicate time to styling the hair to accomplish a desired look, or if they want a wash-and-wear haircut with minimum up-keep. If they are going to change the form of the hair with a permanent wave or a hair straightener, it will be best to give the haircut after the hair has been chemically treated. Also, check the condition of the hair; if the hair is damaged she may want you to cut it shorter to eliminate as much damaged hair as possible.

The form and texture of the hair will determine the appropiate length and haircut:

Best haircuts for straight to wavy hair with thin to medium texture are: one-level, bob, bob variations, bi-level with bobbed back, and wedge haircuts.

Best haircuts for wavy, curly and super-curly hair with medium to thick texture are: one-level, bi-level with long-layered back, and long-layered haircuts.

If the hair has been chemically treated the same haircuts will be acceptable but when cutting it, stretch the hair with less tension to avoid breakage. Also, be gentle when washing it and select products with mild ingredients.

Once the hair is washed, observe the following:

1. Natural part of the hair: Wet the hair, comb it straight to the back and watch it as it naturally parts. When cutting and styling hair with a part on the side, follow the hair's natural movement rather than going against it. Observe that the natural parting connects to the cowlick.

2. Natural direction of the hair: Cowlicks located at the crown give direction to the hair. *See fig. 1.46.* The direction is more noticeable in short hair. Long hair is directed at the base by its growth pattern, but the longer the hair the less direction it will show--it has more weight and bends downward. To check the individual pattern of long hair, lift the hair with a comb (do not stretch or pull the hair), and note its direction one half inch from its base. Also examine the cowlick located at the crown and observe how the hair

grows around it. If the top and side hair tend to go toward the bottom as it's common in straight hair, cut it short enough to reduce the weight and add bounce; if the hair grows toward the back common in wavy hair, leave it long enough to keep it from sticking up when you comb it back. On pages 155-156 you'll find details about how to help give direction to the top hair.

If there is a double cowlick (one next to the other in the crown area), the hair will have more tendency to stick up. Make sure to give the right length to the checkpoint and cut the hair with no tension. If you cut the hair with tension the layers will be uneven due to the different growth patterns in that area. Other cowlicks in hairline areas give direction to the hair of the front, back or sides. *Fig. 1.47.*

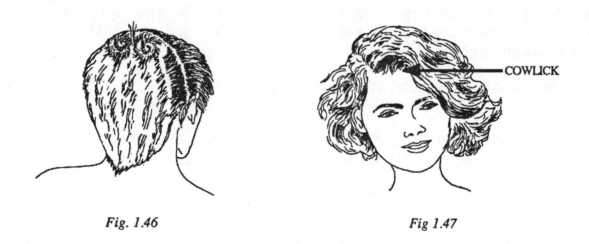

Fig. 1.46   Fig 1.47

The second step is to recommend the appropiate cut to the shape of the face, height, weight and life-style of the person if you wish to obtain the most satisfying haircut. Many people won't care about this factor and only want what they think looks better or feels more comfortable. If that is the case, you will do what the person wants. With experience you will be able to make any length of hair work well with any facial shape.

Observe the person, the face and hairstyle. Visualize the changes that would improve her features. Is the face long or wide? A long face needs some fullness at the sides. Move the hair around, bring it to the sides and observe the effect. Lift the hair in the back. Does a bare neck look better? A wide face needs fullness in the top. Again, move the hair around and observe the different effects accomplished. Make sure that you discuss your observations with the individual.

There are seven major facial shapes:

Oval

Considered to be the perfect shape. You can make a variety of haircuts on an oval shaped face and they will all look good. Through haircutting you will try to bring each facial shape as close to the oval as possible. However, if the person is overweight with an oval face, there will be corrections to be made. According to your observations you may want to cut the hair medium length and give it volume to make the face appear smaller, or leave it long and layer it to make the face appear longer.

Exercise: Use a pencil first to draw the hair around these faces. Once you've drawn a suitable hair design, go over it with a black marker. Visualize what area of the face needs to be covered or be exposed, and where should the head have more or less volume to make the shapes look more attractive. Follow the suggestions indicated for each facial shape, but don't be afraid to get exotic if you want to. This exercise will help you look at faces with a new perspective. I have drawn the hair around the oval shape as a sample. *Fig. 1.48.*

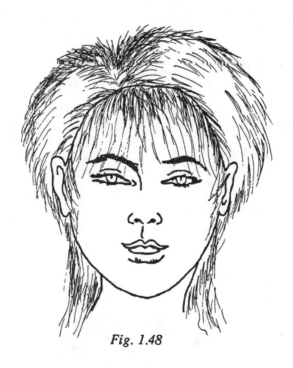

Fig. 1.48

Round

The round face needs to look longer and with less fullness in the cheeks. To correct a round shaped face give volume to the top, leave the sides long over the ears, and bring the hair forward towards the cheeks. Since the round face usually has a short forehead, bangs should be short and layered or no bangs at all. Best haircuts: one-level, bob variation, long-layered. *Fig. 1.49*.

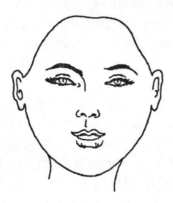

Fig 1.49

<u>Oblong</u>

This face is long and narrow, therefore it needs to look wider and shorter. The hair should be short on top with little volumen and full on the sides. Bangs or a fringe of bangs to camouflage the forehead should make the face appear shorter. The length of the hair should be short to medium (long hair will make the face look longer). Best haircuts: one-level, bob variation, bi-levels (sides with volumen), and wedge. *Fig. 1.50*.

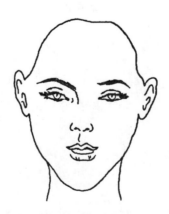

Fig 1.50

Square

The goal is to make the face look longer and to smooth the jawbone. The hairstyle requires fullness on top, bangs or a fringe of bangs, and layers to the sides. The length should cover the structure of the jaw. Best haircuts: long-layered, bob variation, bob with layered top. *Fig. 1.51*.

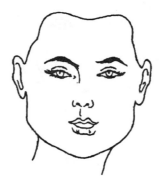

Fig. 1.51

Heart

The forehead is wide, the jaw is narrow and round. The hair should be long to smooth the jaw line. Bangs will help hide a wide forehead. Parting the hair on the side will make the head look less wide on top. Best haircuts: bob, long-layered, bi-levels. *Fig. 1.52*.

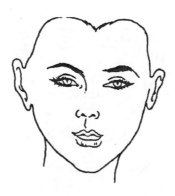

Fig. 1.52

Diamond

The forehead and jawbone are narrow, the cheekbones are high, the overall look of the face is long. The forehead should be covered by bangs or a fringe of bangs, and the cheekbones should be smoothed with hair on the sides. Avoid exposing hairline and ears. Best haircuts: long-layered, one-level, bob variation, wedge. *Fig. 1.53*.

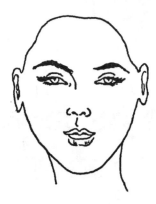

Fig. 1.53

Triangular

The forehead is narrow and the jawbone and chin are wide. You need to make the forehead look wider by giving volumen to the top. The jawbone can be smoothed with hair around the face. Also, a side parting with the hair combed towards the back (avoiding to expose the entire forehead), and short length helps this facial shape look better. Best haircuts: one-level, bob variation, long-layered. *Fig. 1.54*.

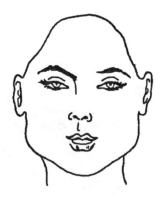

Fig. 1.54

Long hair and flat tops should be avoided if the person is short. Long hair however, suits tall people. Hair that's combed away from the face will accentuate cheekbones and eyes. Towards the face the main focus is on the nose and mouth. These are only general factors to consider. Each person has different characteristics that you must examine and resolve.

Profiles:

When analizing the individual to recommend an appropiate haircut, make sure you also pay attention to her profile. Observe how these have been improved by shaping the hair correctly. The goal is to make the concave and convex look straight. *Fig. 1.55.*

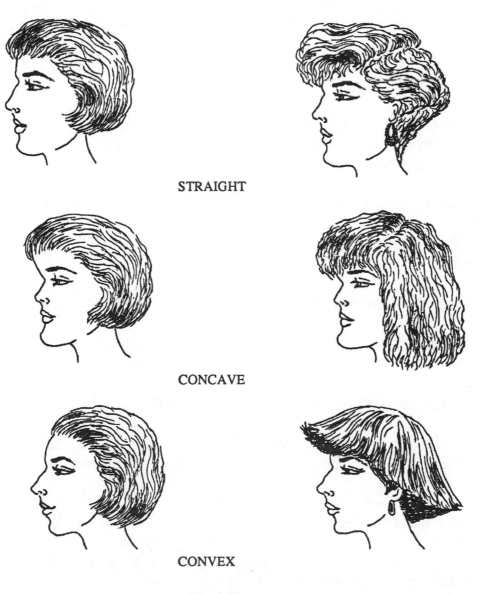

STRAIGHT

CONCAVE

CONVEX

Fig. 1.55

I. BEFORE MAKING THE CUT

Ask the following questions to make sure there is an understanding of what the individual wants, and what you can do to his hair. These questions should be asked before every haircut. Promoting this practice will ensure satisfaction at the end of the haircut. Be sure to memorize them.

1. How long ago was your last haircut and did you like it?

This first question will give you a clue as to how long the hair has grown since the last haircut. If the answer is one month, you can assume that the hair has grown approximately one-half inch, therefore, you'll only trim it. However, if the person did not like it because it was left too long or too short, you'll cut either more or less than one-half inch.

2. How short do you want your length in the back?

Ask the person to show you how much she wants cut. If she has long hair she can bring it forward and show you exactly what she wants cut off. Don't start cutting until you know exactly what the person wants.

3. How short would you like the sides? Above the ear, mid-ear or longer?

Show the length by pointing to your ear and let him show you exactly where he wants his length.

4. How short would you like the top?

Lift the hair at the top with your fingers, look at its length. Does she want the layers short and close to the scalp or does she want fullness?

5. Do you want your hair one-length or layered?

Have her show you where she wants the layers. On the top and sides, on the top only, or all over? Explain what "one-length" means. Make sure you understand how she wants her haircut.

Now that you have clearly established what the subject has in mind in terms of length and style, do not cut it any shorter. In the beginning it is best to be conservative. If you leave the hair longer you can always go back and cut more, but once it is cut too short, only time can correct your error.

Chapter II

TECHNIQUE

Now that you have learned about the tools and the hair, memorized basic terminology, and completed the exercises you are prepared to learn the technique.

To learn a technique is important to every haircutter. It means that you know where to make your guides and how to follow them--the guides will help you blend the layers and shape the hair in the style desired. You will work in a methodical organized way, gradually moving from a starting to an ending point. This method will increase your efficiency, allowing you to complete a perfect haircut in less time.

In this chapter you'll learn how to cut seven different popular haircuts. The primary haircuts are the one-level, the bob and the long-layered. By combining these, other styles are obtained. (The wedge stands on its own.) There are countless variations not included in this book, but with knowledge and practice of this technique, you'll be able to cut them. To be familiar with the looks of each style, see their picture and read their description in the corresponding page for that haircut. The haircuts are: one-level (Section C, page 65); bob (Section D, page 76); bob variation (Section E, page 93); bi-level with bobbed back (Section F, page 101); bi-level with long-layered back (Section G, page 113); long-layered (Section H, page 126); and wedge (Section I, page 139).

These haircuts are composed of four major steps:

1. Parting the hair is the first step. All the sample styles are parted in the same fashion except for the back of the head. The back is parted in three different ways depending on whether the hair is to be one-length, be layered, or be a wedge haircut.

2. The outline or perimeter is the second step. The outline will be started and ended the same way for all haircuts. You'll only change the length of the outline at different points around the head according to the style to be cut.

3. Layering is the third step. There are three methods to make layers, (1) for short hair, (2) for long hair, and (3) for the wedge haircut. One-length haircuts do not require this step.

4. Checking is the fourth and last step. There are three methods: (1) for short layers, (2) for long layers, and (3) for one-length haircuts.

To memorize the steps of each haircut there are several methods you can t r y : 1) Answer the questions at the end of each Section, if there is something you forgot look it up. 2) Review the technique and jot down the steps of each haircut after reading the book. 3) Read the technique and have a friend ask you to list the steps to each haircut making sure you don't miss any. 4) Record the steps to the haircuts in a tape player and listen to it several times. 5) Watch the videotape "Haircutting Basics" (refer to the Appendix for information on how to obtain it). With this videotape you will learn the steps quickly. The goal is to be able to automatically follow the steps from beginning to end so you can fully concentrate on following your guides and creating the desired look.

Now, read carefully the steps to follow and get a clear understanding of the haircutting technique before you start the actual cutting. Afterwards you may wish to practice on a friend or a wig.

A. PARTING THE HAIR

Parting the hair refers to the division of the hair into main portions. It is important to distribute the hair to organize your sections and guides as required by the size of the head, bone structure and intended hair design.

Before the hair is parted it should be washed and untangled. Be sure to maintain the hair wet thorought the haircut.

One-level, bi-level with long-layered back, long-layered and wedge haircuts should be parted as explained below. To part a bob, a bi-level with bobbed back and a bob variation, see Section D, pages 77-78.

1. Top parting: center, from the crown to the forehead. *Fig. 2.1*.

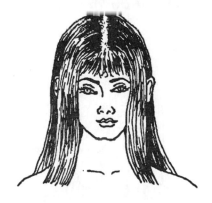

Fig. 2.1

2. Side parting: from ear-to-ear. *Fig. 2.2*.

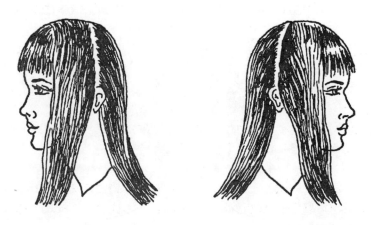

Fig. 2.2

3. Front parting: triangle, from one-third of the top to the temples. *Fig. 2.3*.

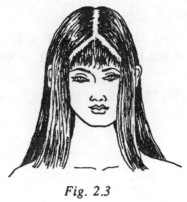

Fig. 2.3.

4. Back:

a) Layered cuts: smooth the hair down with no partings. *Fig. 2.4*.

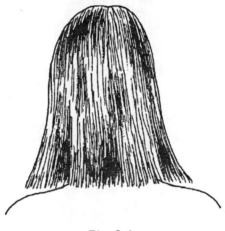

Fig. 2.4

b) Wedge: make V parting from the top of the ears to the occipital bone. *Fig. 2.5*.

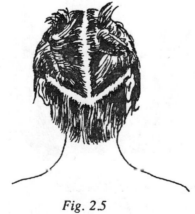

Fig. 2.5

B. THE OUTLINE

The outline is the perimeter that serves as an edge to define the surrounding lengths of the haircut. This edge can have any shape or length desired. The outline is always cut at **zero** elevation.

The outline is composed of four areas: (1) back, (2) front, (3) left side, (4) right side. Eventually you'll be cutting it with the hair flat on the skin. Now, to avoid accidental cuts, place the hair between your fingers and stretch it at zero elevation. Cut with the scissors close to the fingers on the palm side of your hand.

Note: To outline a bob and bob variation see page 76.
To outline a bi-level with bobbed back see page 101.

a) To Outline the Back: one-level, bi-level with long-layered back, long-layered and wedge.

<u>From the center of the back to the left side</u>

1. After discussing with the subject the desired length and hairstyle, part the hair accordingly. See illustrations in Section A, pages 51-52.

2. Tilt the subject's head forward to avoid tapering the outline and to have a comfortable position for cutting. If you are outlining a wedge make sure the hair is short. If the hair is below the nape the ends will flip up.

3. Comb the hair of the back free of tangles.

4. Hold a one-inch wide section of hair from the center of the back. Slide your fingers to the point where you want to cut. Keep the fingers near the blades to cut in a straight line. *Fig. 2.6.*

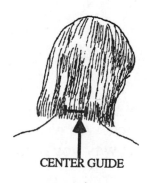

CENTER GUIDE

Fig. 2.6

5. Cut toward the left side in small snips with the tips of the scissors. Do not cut beyond the second joint of the index finger. Only the hair stretched between the first two joints pulls the hair with even tension.

6. Snip five times, stop comb; make a new section and include one-quarter inch of the section previously cut as a guide to the length. Do not cut the guide, only continue extending the line from the center.

7. Cut slowly and stand back at times to observe how is your outline coming along.

8. Once you cut the left side of the back in a straight line, comb the hair again, go back to the starting point, and check if your line is straight and clean; if it is not, cut where needed only. Do not cut the hair shorter than you had planned. If your line is not perfectly straight leave it as it is or you may cut it too short. With practice your line will be perfect. *Fig. 2.7.*

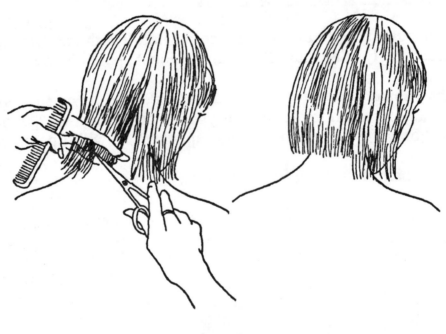

Fig. 2.7

Now, the left side of the back outline is completed. Breath deeply and get ready to start cutting the right side of the back. An easy and accurate method to cut it is by breaking the line in two sections. This way you'll have the guide visible at all times as explained in the proceeding steps.

<u>From the center of the back to the right side</u>

1. Tilt the subject's head forward.

2. Start in the middle of the right section and cut towards the center. *Fig. 2.8.*

3. Cut section two and join it with section one. *Fig. 2.9.*

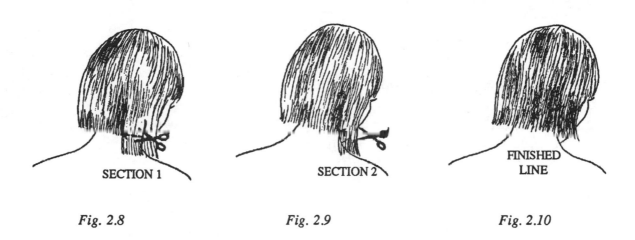

SECTION 1   SECTION 2   FINISHED
                                         LINE

Fig. 2.8   *Fig. 2.9*   *Fig. 2.10*

b) To Outline the Front

The front outline may have any shape you want. It can be made straight, or angled (longer in the middle or shorter in the middle). In the sample haircut I'll explain how to cut the front outline shorter in the middle. *Fig. 2.11.*

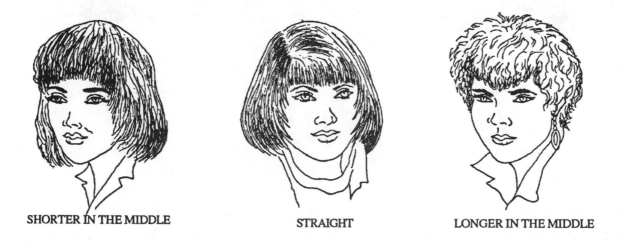

SHORTER IN THE MIDDLE   STRAIGHT   LONGER IN THE MIDDLE

Fig. 2.11

55

Usually eyebrow level or longer is a good length for the front outline. Remember that cowlicks and widow's peaks are common in the front hairline, so keep an eye for them.

From the center of the front to the right temple

1. Lift the subject's head straight.

2. Stand in front of the subject.

3. Re-adjust the front parting.

4. Cut a center guide on top of the nose. *Fig. 2.12*.

5. Cut from the center guide to the right temple in a downward direction. *Fig. 2.13*. To give extra length to the front hair, cut below the temple.

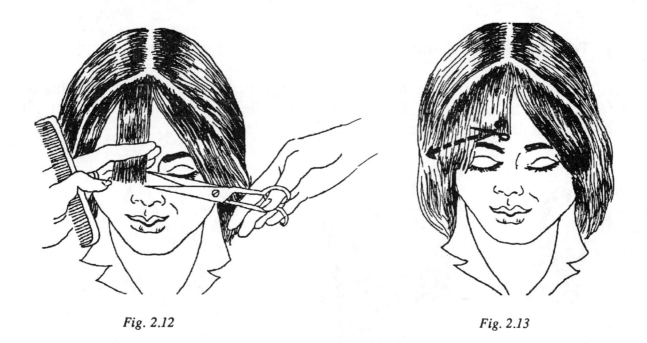

Fig. 2.12   Fig. 2.13

Now the right side is completed. Breath deeply and get ready to cut the left side.

From the center of the front to the left temple

The left side of the front outline will be parted in two sections. This way you'll always have your guide visible.

1. Cut the first section and join it with the center guide. *Fig. 2.14.*

2. Cut the second section in an upward direction from the left temple to section one and join them. Make sure that you place your fingers in the same angle you had them on the right side. *Fig. 2.15.*

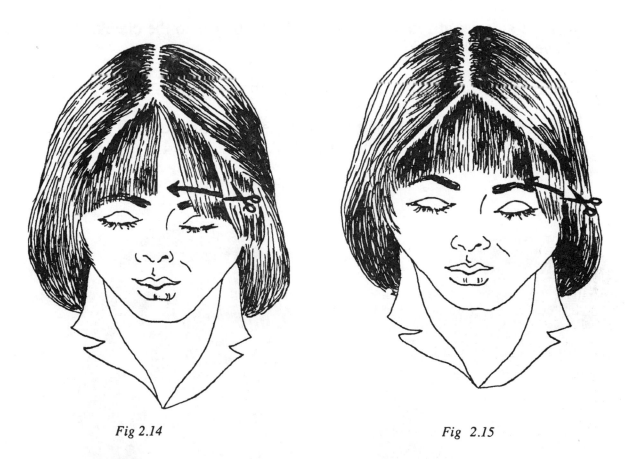

Fig 2.14   Fig 2.15

3. Once the left side is finished stand back and observe. Make the necessary adjustments.

Do you have an even curvature? Is the hair too short, too long? If the hair is too long make a new guide in the center and start again. Adjustments should be made cutting one-quarter inch at a time. Remember that once the hair dries it will be shorter.

To outline the sides of a long-layered haircut, turn to page 60.

c) To Outline the Sides: short hair (one-level, bi-level, wedge).

<u>Left Side</u>

1. Stand next to the subject's left side.

2. Re-establish ear-to-ear parting.

3. Tilt the subject's head to the right side.

4. Comb the hair down over the ear. *Fig. 2.16.*

5. Cut the side length in a straight line from the ear to the cheek. Do not cut above the hairline. *Fig. 2.16.*

6. Comb all the hair of the left side towards the front. *Fig. 2.17.*

7. Cut in an upward direction toward the temple and meet the frontal outline. Make sure to drop the outline. *Fig. 2.17.*

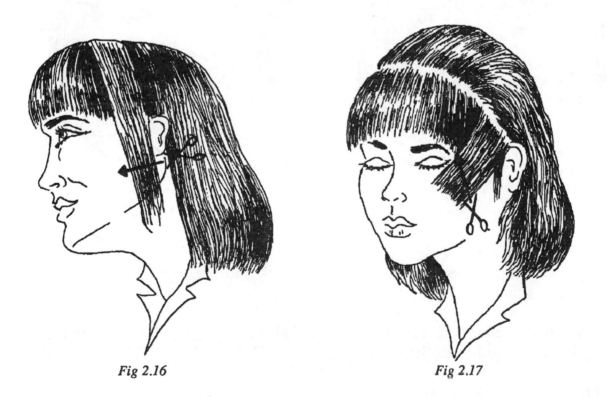

Fig 2.16   *Fig 2.17*

Now the left side is completed. Get ready to cut the right side.

Right Side

Proceed to outline the right side using the same method.

1. Stand next to the subject's right side.

2. Re-adjust ear-to-ear parting.

3. Tilt the subject's head to the left side.

4. Comb the hair over the ear. *Fig. 2.18.*

5. Cut the same length of the left side. You may use the bones of the ears as points of reference to make sure that both sides have the same length. *Fig. 2.18.*

6. Comb the hair of the right side toward the front. *Fig. 2.19.*

7. Cut in a downward direction from the right temple to the earlobe. *Fig. 2.19.*

8. Breath deeply; stand back and observe.

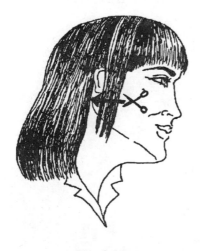

Fig. 2.18

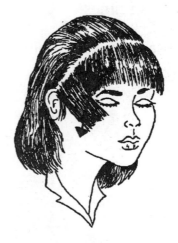

Fig 2.19

Now both sides are completed. To continue and finish the haircuts listed below, return to their corresponding Section and page.

One-level: Section C, page 68. Bi-level with long-layered back: Section G, page 117. Wedge: Section I, page 143.

d) To Outline the Sides: long hair (long-layered, bob variation).

1. If the hair of the sides is below the shoulders and the style is straight, turn the head to the left and align chin over shoulder. Cut the side using the back length as a guide. Cut from the back to the left side. *Fig. 2.20.*

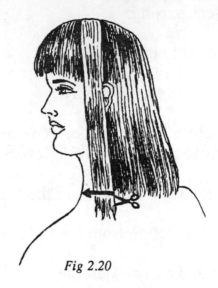

Fig 2.20

To cut the right side, first divide it in two sections; this way you'll have the guide visible at all times.

1. Cut section one to join with the back. *Fig. 2.21.*

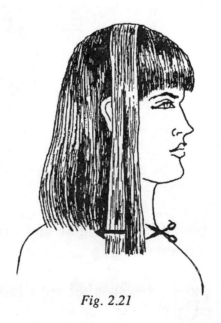

Fig. 2.21

2. Cut section two from the front to section one. *Fig. 2.22.*

3. To check that both sides have equal lengths tilt the head forward and measure with the comb, or meet the ends of the sides in the front. See illustrations on page 63.

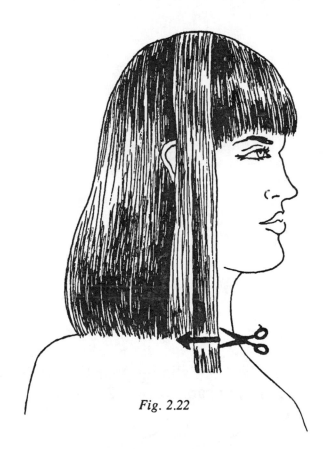

Fig. 2.22

e)   To Angle the Sides of Long Hair   (long-layered, bob variation).

If the hair of the sides is long and to be layered, such as in a bob variation or a long-layered haircut, they may be angled to give graduation to the outline; the result will be a feathery effect on the sides and more movement of the side hair towards the back.

Cut the sides as explained above in Section (d) and proceed as follows:

Place your hand in the angle that you want to cut. Use the bones or features of the face as a guide to the length. If the hair is very long you may want to use other parts of the body as a reference to the length.

Left Side

1. Stand facing the subject's left side.

2. Elevate the hair sliding the fingers towards the front. Let outline drop.

3. Cut on the palm side of your hand. *Fig. 2.23.*

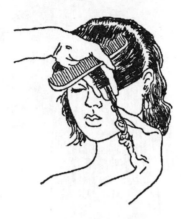

Fig 2.23

Right side

1. Stand behind the subject.

2. Lift the hair towards the front sliding your fingers in vertical position, and cut on the back side of your hand. *Fig. 2.24.*

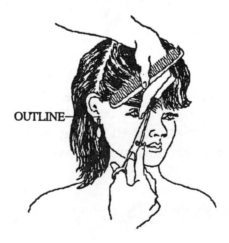

OUTLINE

Fig. 2.24

Now the sides have been angled. Check the lengths as follows:

Tilt the head forward and let the hair of the sides hang. With the comb parallel to the floor measure the sides and make sure they are the same length. *Fig. 2.25.*

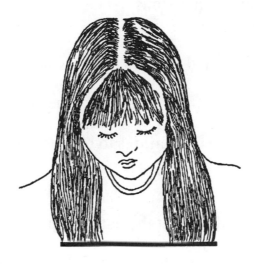

Fig 2.25

Another way to measure the sides is by meeting the side lengths in the front. *Fig. 2.26.*

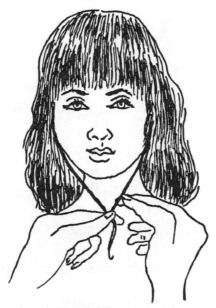

Fig. 2.26

Now the outline is finished. To complete a bob variation, return to Section E, page 96. To complete a long-layered haircut return to Section H, page 130.

REVIEW QUESTIONS

To make sure that you thoroughly understand the steps necessary to cut the outline, answer the following questions. The answers can be found in the page numbers noted at the side.

1. How do the eyebrows and temples help you cut the front outline? pp. 35-36

2. What are some of the different lengths of the side outline? p. 37

3. What would determine the partings to be made before outlining the hair? p. 51

4. What is an outline? p. 53

5. At what degree would you cut the outline? p. 53

6. Where would you start the outline? p. 53

7. What are the three other areas that compose an outline and in what order are they cut? p. 53

8. Why should the head be tilted forward or to the side, when the hair is being outlined? p. 53

9. List the sections of the back outline. p. 53

10. List the guides that help you cut the back outline. pp. 53, 55

11. List the sections of the front outline. pp. 56-57

12. List the sections of the left side short outline. p. 58

13. What styles have a short outline on the sides? p. 58

14. List the sections of the right side of a short outline. p. 59

15. How would you outline the sides of long hair? pp. 60-61

16. How would you angle the sides of long hair? pp. 60-62

17. What styles with long hair have angled sides? p. 61

C. ONE-LEVEL

The one-level haircut is an easy-care style, a favorite of many women of all ages and a man's classic haircut.

This style can be cut super short or longer. The layers can be shaped to provide volume to the top and length to the back, while the sides can be tapered close to the head. Another variation is with the top long and the sides and the back very short; also, you can keep it short all over framing the face. Just be aware that with the same basic technique, you can accomplish many different looks by adjusting the length of the layers in different areas of the head. *Fig. 2.27.*

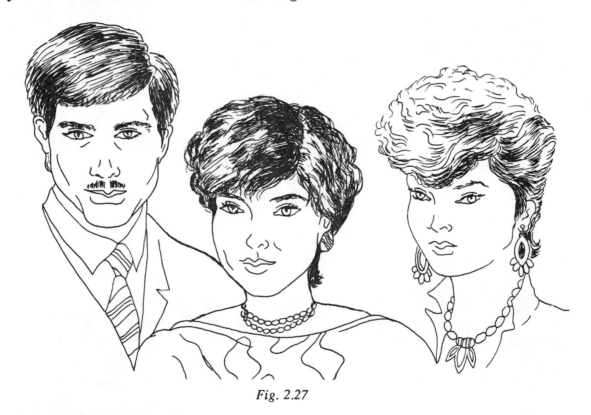

Fig. 2.27

PARTING THE HAIR

See illustrations on Section A, page 51.

Top parting: center, from the crown to the forehead.

Side parting: from ear-to-ear.

Front parting: triangle, from one-third of the top to the temples.

Back: smooth it down with no parting.

GUIDES

The following guides will be used to cut a one-level haircut.

Hairline
Top of the nose
Eyebrows   }   OUTLINE
Ears
Perimeter

Crown-level checkpoint
Nose   }   LAYERS
Top section
Sections and layers

ANGLES

This style will be cut at a ninety-degree angle. *Fig. 2.28.*

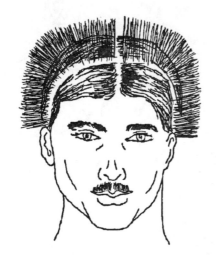 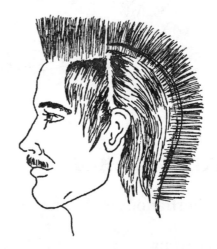

Fig 2.28

LAYERED SECTIONS

Adjust the number of sections according to the size of the head.

Section one corresponds to the top. *Fig. 2.29.*

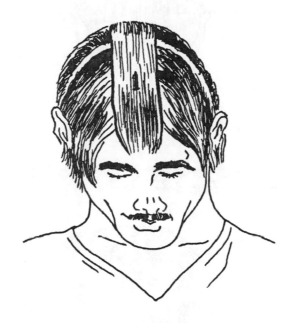

Fig. 2.29

Section two, left side. *Fig. 2.30.*

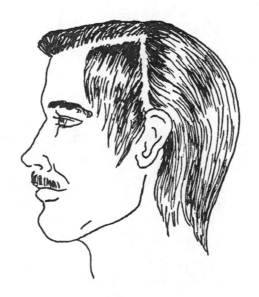

Fig. 2.30

Sections three, four, five, six and seven, to the back. *Fig. 2.31.*

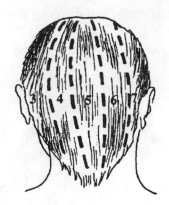

Fig. 2.31

Section eight, right side. *Fig. 2.32.*

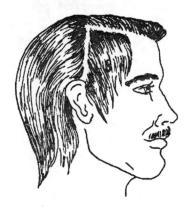

Fig. 2.32

OUTLINE

1. Outline the back, front and sides. See page 53 for details.

Once the outline is completed, return to this page and proceed to cut the layers as follows:

CUTTING THE LAYERS

Section One: top

1. Stand next to the subject's left side.

2. Cut crown-level checkpoint. See page 34 for details to cut this guide.

3. Comb the top hair forward. *Fig. 2.33*.

4. Make a two-inch wide section from crown-level checkpoint to the front. *Fig. 2.33*.

5. Elevate one-third of the section at a time at a ninety-degree angle. Use the nose as a guide to center section one. *Fig. 2.34*.

6. Cut from crown-level checkpoint to the front perimeter in a straight line. Let the front perimeter drop. *Fig. 2.34*.

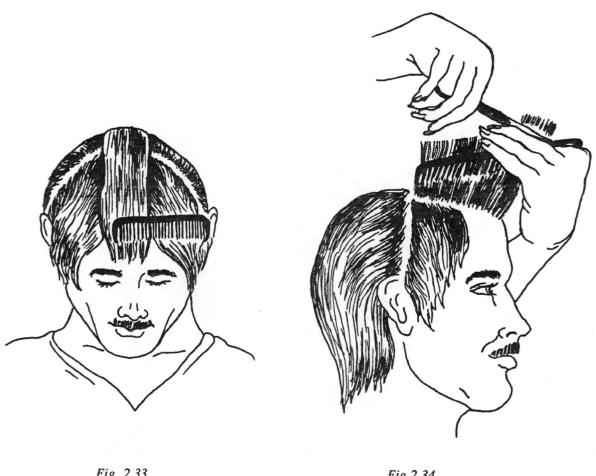

Fig. 2.33   Fig 2.34

Now the top has been completed, breath deeply and get ready to layer the sides.

Section Two: left side

1. Remain next to the subject's left side. Make a center parting in the the top and re-adjust ear-to-ear parting.

2. Make a straight and vertical side section from the ear to the top.

3. Elevate the perimeter at a ninety-degree angle and use it as the first guide to the length of the layers. Cut this section in vertical direction from the perimeter to the top. *Fig. 2.35.*

4. Snip five times, drop the hair, comb it, take more hair, elevate it and cut again. Always use a one-quarter inch of the layers previously cut as a guide to the length of the next section.

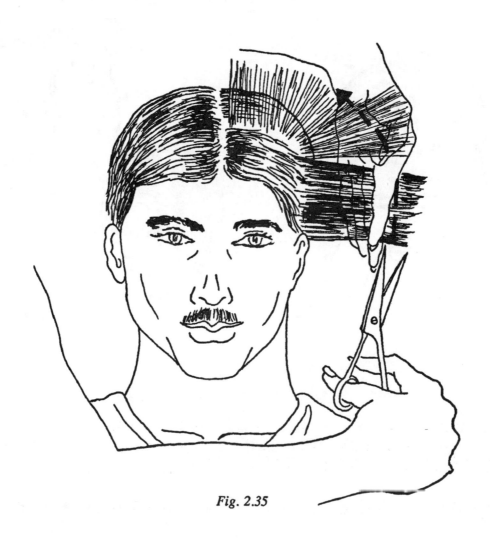

Fig. 2.35

Section Three thru Seven: back

You will need to make more or less sections according to the size of the head. A child's head is smaller than an adult's and since children grow very impatient in a short period of time you need to finish the haircut as fast as you can, therefore, three sections may be enough to cut the layers of the back. A large head however, may need more than five sections. Make adjustments as necessary.

1. Stand next to the subject's left side and move around the back as you approach the left side.

2. Make clean vertical sections, one-and-a-half to two inches wide. Include one-quarter inch from previous sections as a guide to the length.

3. Starting at the hairline elevate the hair at a ninety-degree angle and cut upwards to join the side with the top. *Fig. 2.36.*

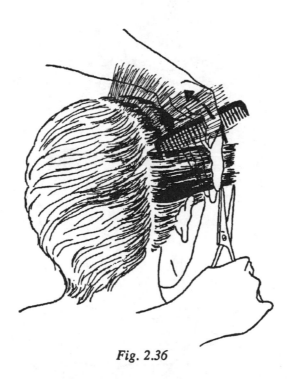

Fig. 2.36

Make sure that your guide is visible at all times with each new section you hold. If you lose your guide stop, define your section and then continue, or bend the ends of the hair as you hold it to see the length of your guide.

4. Repeat the steps adding sections until you get to section eight on the right side.

Section Eight: right side

1. Re-adjust ear-to-ear parting.

2. Stand behind the subject's right shoulder. In this position you should be able to see your guide.

3. Make a section from the ear to the front. Include one-quarter inch of section eight as a guide to the length.

4. Cut from the perimeter to the top. When you elevate section eight do not stretch the hair towards the back. Make sure you are holding the hair at a ninety-degree angle, otherwise this section will be longer than section two on the left side of the head. *Fig. 2.37.*

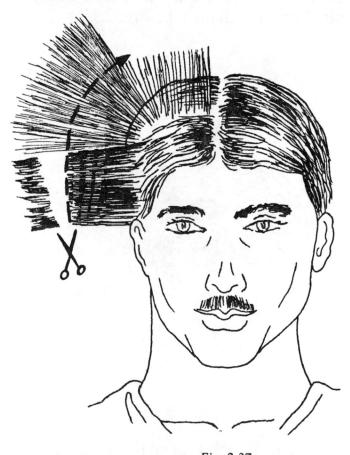

Fig. 2.37

5. Breath deeply; stand back, observe and get ready to check the haircut.

CHECKING

Once you have cut the last section, the next step is to check the haircut. If the sections are uneven, even them out. Do not make unnecessary cuts and do not make new guides.

Ask yourself if you have made any of the following mistakes; they could be the reasons to uneven lengths of hair in your sections: Did you apply too much tension to some sections? Did you stretch the hair with tension in the cowlick areas? Did you follow the guide at all times? Were some of the sections too large and others too small? Did you make clean partings?

Stand behind the subject and start checking the hair in the following way:

1. Crown: Take a horizontal section at the crown, elevate it at a ninety-degree angle. Ideally this section should be perfectly straight. If it is longer on one side, it indicates that one side of the head has longer hair. In this case start the haircut from the beginning. Otherwise even out the hair and go on to the next step. *Fig. 2.38*.

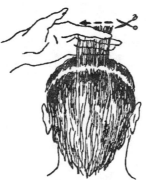

Fig. 2.38

2. Top: Make a section on top and stand behind the subject. Check the hair at a ninety-degree angle in three horizontal sections from the crown to the front. *Fig. 2.39*.

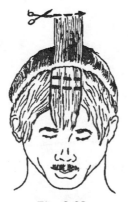

Fig. 2.39

73

3. Sides: Check the sides horizontally starting at the top and working your way down to the hairline. Hold the hair at a ninety-degree angle and cut if necessary to even out the hair. *Fig. 2.40*.

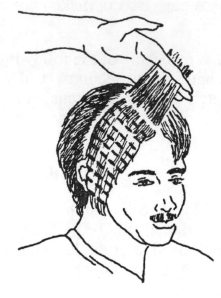

Fig. 2.40

4. Back: Elevate the hair of the crown at a ninety-degree angle. Continue checking the center of the back in horizontal sections until you reach the perimeter. Do the left and the right side of the back from the top to the perimeter. *Fig. 2.41*. If there is hair flipping up behind the ears, comb the hair forward and cut the ends extending beyond the hairline. *Fig. 2.42*.

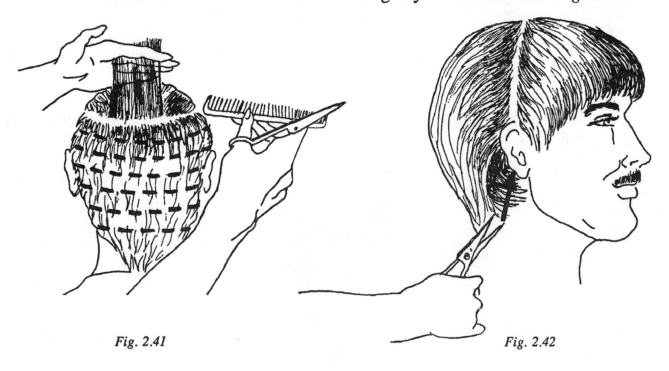

Fig. 2.41   *Fig. 2.42*

REVIEW QUESTIONS

To ensure that you have learned the steps of the one-level haircut, answer the following questions. The page numbers next to the questions indicate where the answers can be found.

1. How can the perimeter be a guide? p. 33

2. Explain what each of the following guides indicate: pp. 32-39
   a) hairline
   b) crown-level checkpoint
   c) nose
   d) top section
   e) sections and layers

3. Why can the crown present problems? p. 42

4. What are the five questions to ask before starting the haircut? p. 48

5. How would you part the hair to cut a one-level style? p. 65

6. At what degree would you elevate the hair to cut a one-level? p. 66

7. List the sections of the one-level haircut. pp. 67-68

8. What would you cut first, the outline or the layers? pg 68

9. Where would you start layering the hair and where would you end the haircut? pp. 69-74

10. In what direction (vertical or horizontal), would you cut side and back layers? p. 70

11. Explain briefly how would you check the top, back and sides of this haircut. pp. 73-74

12. In what direction would you hold the hair to check it, vertically or horizontally? pp. 73-74

D. BOB

The bob haircut is a one-length hairstyle excellent for straight hair that needs bounce. Most popular manageable lengths range from jawbone to just above the shoulders. These lengths allow the bob freedom of movement for a bouncy look and its line will not be disturbed by the hair touching the shoulders. *Fig. 2.43.*

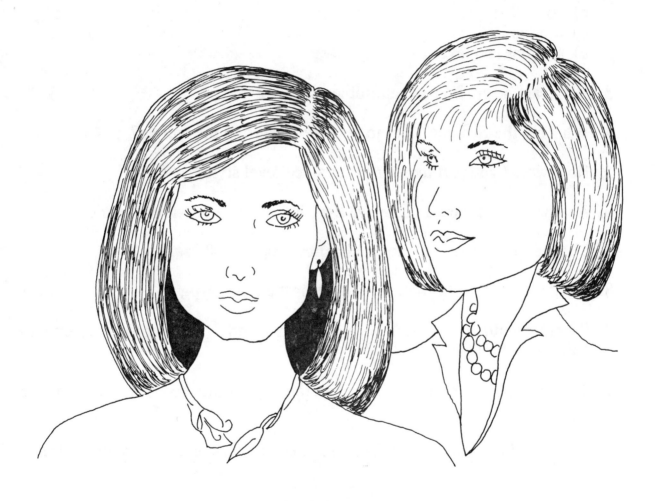

Fig. 2.43

PARTING THE HAIR

Top parting: center, from the crown to the forehead. *Fig. 2.44.*

Some people wear this style with a side parting. If the person is going to wear it parted on the side all the time, you must cut it parted on that side; this way, the hair of the top will have the length of the side perimeter. *Fig. 2.45.*

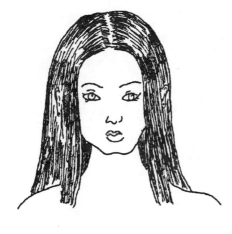

Fig 2.44

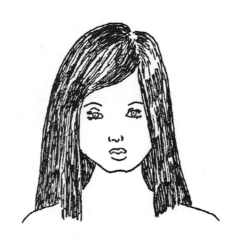

Fig 2.45

Side parting: from ear-to-ear. *Fig. 2.46.*

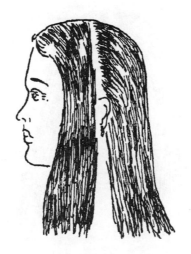

Fig. 2.46

If the hair is very thick, divide the hair in half-horizontals in the following way:

Make a horizontal parting at eye level from ear-to-ear parting to the front. Pin the upper section out of the way and smooth the rest of the hair down. *Fig. 2.47.*

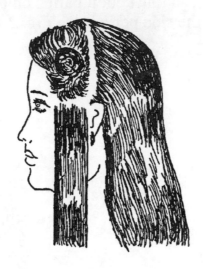

Fig. 2.47

Front parting: for bangs, make triangle parting from one-third of the top to the temples. *Fig. 2.48.*

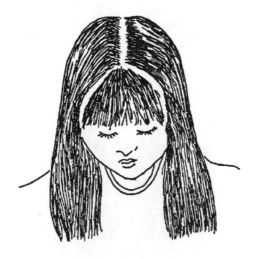

Fig. 2.48

Back parting: triangle, from the occipital bone to below the ears. Pin the upper section out of the way and smooth the rest of the hair down. *Fig. 2.49.*

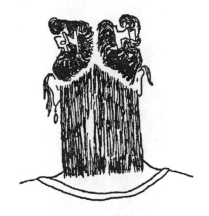

Fig. 2.49

GUIDES

Shoulders
Top of the nose
Back perimeter
Eyebrows
Temples
Sections

ANGLES

The bob is cut at zero elevation. *Fig. 2.50.*

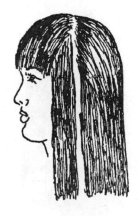

Fig. 2.50

SECTIONS

Sections one, two and three correspond to the first layer of the back. *Fig. 2.51.*

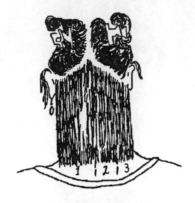

Fig. 2.51

Sections four, five and six to the second layer of the back. *Fig. 2.52.*

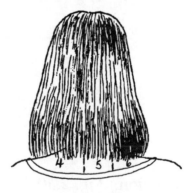

Fig. 2.52

Section seven, left side. *Fig. 2.53.*

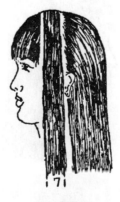

Fig. 2.53

Section eight and nine, right side. *Fig. 2.54.*

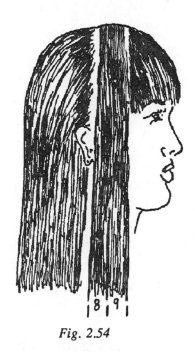

Fig. 2.54.

Sections ten, eleven and twelve, bangs. *Fig. 2.55.*

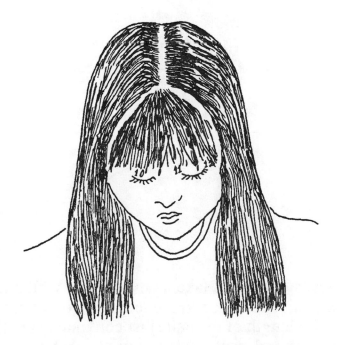

Fig. 2.55

CUTTING THE SECTIONS

BACK

**First Layer of the Back
Section One: left side**

1. Part the hair.

2. Stand behind the subject.

3. Tilt the subject's head forward, and ask her to keep it that way while you cut the back to avoid taper in the perimeter.

4. Place a one-inch wide section from the center of the back between the middle and index fingers of your left hand. Slide your fingers to the point where you want to cut. Keep the scissors close to the fingers to keep the line straight.

5. Cut toward the left side in small snips with the tips of the scissors. *Fig. 2.56.* Do not cut beyond the second joint of the index finger, this way you will avoid accidental cuts to your hand and the perimeter will be straight.

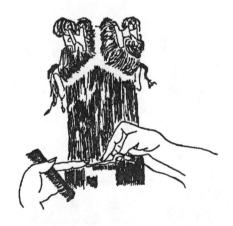

Fig. 2.56

6. Snip five times, stop, comb, take a new section with one-quarter inch of the hair previously cut as a guide to the length. Do not cut the guide, if you do you'll change the length of the hair; just continue extending the line from the center. Cut slowly and stand back at times to observe.

7. Once you have cut the left side in a straight line, comb the hair again, go back to the starting point, and check if your line is straight and clean. If it is not, cut where needed only.

Do not cut the hair shorter than planned. If your line is not perfectly straight leave it as it is or you may cut it too short. With practice, your lines will be perfect.

Now the left side of the back outline is completed. Breath deeply and get ready to cut the right side of the back outline as explained below:

Sections Two and Three: right side

An easy accurate method to cut the right side is by breaking the perimeter in two sections. This way you will have the guide visible at all times.

1. Tilt the subject's head forward.

2. Start in the middle of the right side.

3. Cut section two towards the center guide. *Fig. 2.57.*

4. Move to section three and cut to join it with section two. *Fig. 2.58.*

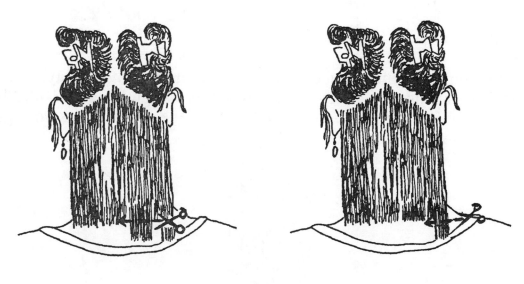

Fig. 2.57   Fig. 2.58

Now the back is completed. Get a mirror and show the back length to the person. Make sure this is the length desired. If it's too long make a new guide and cut more, otherwise check the back as follows:

5. Gather the hair in your comb and slide it down from the parting to the perimeter. Place the comb parallel to the floor and check the line. If there are a few wisps of hair hanging, cut them. If the crooked areas are less than one-quarter inch too long, leave the length alone. If there are differences in length of one-half inch or more start from the beginning with a new guide. *Fig. 2.59.*

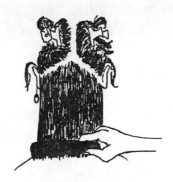

Fig. 2.59

Second Layer of the Back
Section Four: left side

1. Once the first layer of the back is completed bring the rest of the hair down and comb it free of tangles.

2. Tilt the subject's head forward.

3. Cut from the center to the left as you did in the previous layer. This time, roll your fingers down to make this layer slightly longer--the hair will naturally fold under. Follow the length of the first layer as your guide, but make sure you are not cutting it. *Fig. 2.60.*

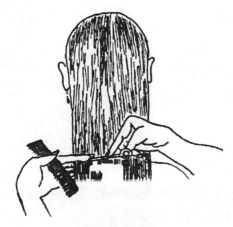

Fig. 2.60

Sections Five and Six: right side

1. Divide the right side in two sections. Use the same procedure of the first layer, but this time, roll the fingers down as indicated in section four.

2. Cut section five and join it to section four. *Fig. 2.61.*

3. Cut from section six to section five and join those two sections. *Fig. 2.62.*

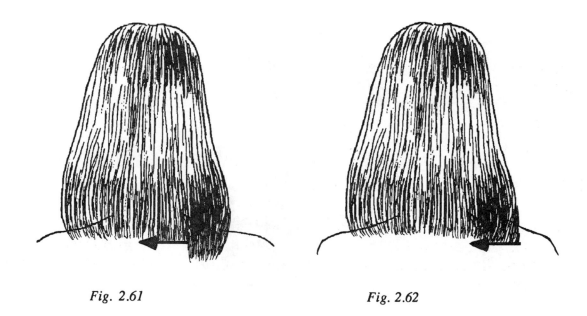

Fig. 2.61   Fig. 2.62

Now the back has been completed. If you are cutting a bi-level with bobbed back, you can now return to Section F, page 108 to complete the haircut. If you are cutting a bob proceed to the next page to cut the sides.

SIDES.
Section Seven: left side

If the sides had thick abundant hair and were parted in half-horizontals, cut the first layer straight and the second layer rolling the fingers down. Otherwise do not roll the fingers to cut the sides. Also if you are cutting a bob variation you don't need to roll the fingers down.

1. Move to the subject's left side.

2. Roll the fingers down while you hold the hair and continue cutting the outline towards the left side. *Fig. 2.63*.

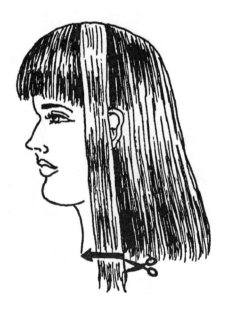

Fig. 2.63

Sections Eight and Nine: right side

1. Stand next to the subject's right side.

An easy accurate method to cut the right side is by breaking the line in two sections to have your guide visible.

2. Cut section eight and join it to the back. *Fig. 2.64*.

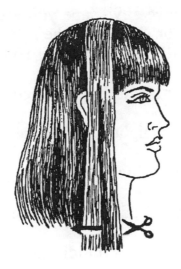

Fig. 2.64

3. Cut section nine from the front to section eight. Stretch the hair at zero elevation while you cut. *Fig. 2.65*.

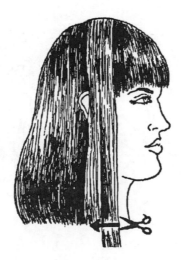

Fig. 2.65

Now the sides are completed. Breath deeply and get ready to cut the front.

FRONT
Section Ten: right side

The front outline may have any shape you want. It can be made straight, or angled (longer in the middle or shorter in the middle). In the sample haircut I'll explain how to cut the front outline shorter in the middle.

Usually, eyebrow level or longer is a good length for the front outline.

1. Lift the subject's head straight, and face the subject.

2. Re-adjust the triangle parting on the front.

3. Hold a one-inch strand of hair in the middle of the forehead.

4. Cut it at zero elevation. This middle strand will be a guide to the length of the front outline. *Fig. 2.66.*

5. Cut section ten from top of the nose to the below the temple in a downward direction. *Fig. 2.67.*

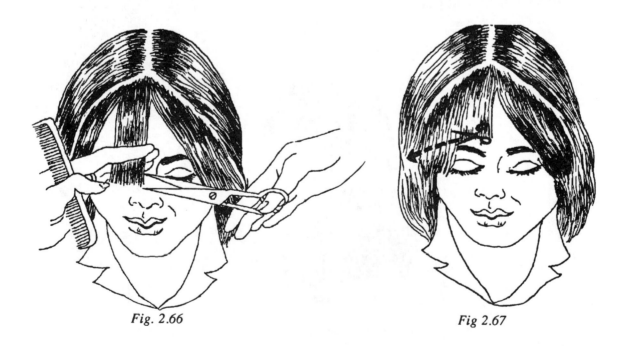

Fig. 2.66   Fig 2.67

Now the right side is completed. Check that the line is straight and get ready to cut the left side.

Sections Eleven and Twelve: left side

The left side of the front outline will be parted in two sections. This way you'll always have your guide visible.

1. Cut section eleven at zero elevation and join it with the center guide. *Fig. 2.68.*

2. Cut section twelve in an upward direction, from the left temple to section eleven, and join both sections. *Fig. 2.69.*

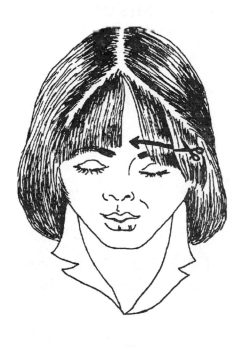

Fig. 2.68

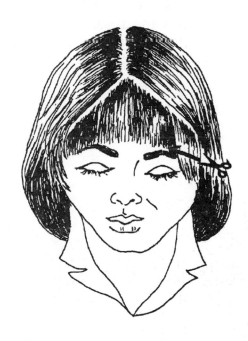

Fig. 2.69

3. Breath deeply; stand back and observe.

Note: To angle the sides of a bob variation turn to Section B, page 62.

CHECKING

Once you have cut the last section, the next step is to check the haircut. If there is uneven hair in the sections, cut them even. Do not make unnecessary cuts and do not make new guides.

Ask yourself if you have made any of the following mistakes; they could be the reasons to uneven lengths of hair in your sections: Did you apply too much tension to some sections of hair? Did you follow the guide at all times? Did you maintain the scissors straight with your fingers? Did you tilt the head forward while cutting the back? Did you cut the hair at zero elevation at all times? Now, stand behind the subject and check the haircut in the following way.

1. Back: Gather the hair of the back in your comb and slide it down from the occipital bone to the perimeter. Place the comb parallel to the floor and check the line. If the perimeter is uneven, cut where the lengths are longer. If the length is one-half inch longer on one side, part the hair and start from the beginning. *Fig. 2.70.*

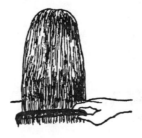

Fig. 2.70

2. Sides: Tilt the subject's head forward and allow the sides to hang. Use your comb to measure that they are equally long, or meet the ends in the front. *Fig. 2.71.*

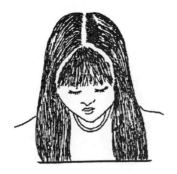
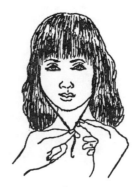

Fig 2.71

Note: To layer the bangs turn to Chapter III, page 153.

How to Cut a One Level Top on a Bob Haircut

1. Part the hair from ear-to-ear.

2. Cut top-level checkpoint. See page 34 for details.

3. Make a triangle section from top-level checkpoint to the temples. *Fig. 2.72.*

4. Elevate the section at a ninety-degree angle in a vertical direction. *Fig. 2.73.*

5. Cut from the checkpoint to the front. Make sure the perimeter drops uncut. *Fig. 2.73.*

6. Stand behind the subject.

7. Check the hair in three horizontal sections from the checkpoint to the front. *Fig. 2.74.*

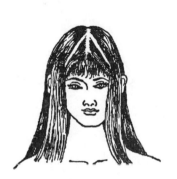

Fig. 2.72

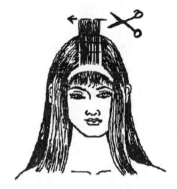

Fig. 2.74

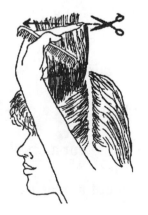

Fig. 2.73

REVIEW QUESTIONS

To ensure that you have learned the steps of the bob haircut, answer the following questions. The page numbers next to the questions indicate where the answers can be found.

1. Explain how the following guides help you cut a bob. pp. 32-39
   a) Shoulders   d) Eyebrows
   e) Temples   b) Back perimeter
   f) Sections   c) Top of the nose

2. How would you part the hair to cut a bob? pp. 77-78

3. How would you cut the hair if the person always parts her hair on the side? p. 77

4. What are half-horizontals? p. 78

5. At what degree would you cut a bob? p. 79

6. Why is it important not to cut into the guides? p. 82

7. Why is it important to tilt the head forward while cutting the back. p. 82

8. Where would you start cutting the sections? p. 82

9. What's an accurate way to cut the right side of the back? p. 83

10. How would you place your fingers to cut the second layer? p. 84

11 Where would you start cutting the front and in how many sections? pp. 88-89

12. Where would you end the haircut? p. 90

13. How would you part the hair to cut a one-level top? p. 91

14. What guides would you use to cut a one-level top? p. 91

15. At what degree would you cut a one-level top? p. 91

16. In what direction would you check a one-level top? p. 91

E. BOB VARIATION--bob with one-level top and long-layered sides

This haircut combines three styles. The back is one-length, the sides are long and layered, the top is short and layered. The layers of the top and sides will bring bounce and volume to wavy hair or a feathered look to straight hair. Through styling, this haircut can be changed into a number of different looks to match a variety of daytime or evening activities. *Fig. 2.75.*

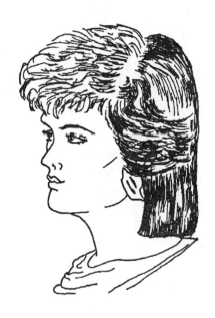

Fig. 2.75

PARTING THE HAIR

Part the hair for a bob. Illustrations are on page 77.

Top parting: center, from the crown to the front.

Side parting: from ear-to-ear.

Front parting: triangle, from one-third of the top to the temples.

Back parting: triangle, from occipital bone to below the ears. Pin the upper section out of the way, and smooth the rest of the hair down.

GUIDES

Back perimeter
Top of the nose   }   OUTLINE
Temples
Eyebrows

Top-level checkpoint
Nose   }   LAYERS
Top section
Sections and layers

ANGLES

Top: ninety-degree angle. *Fig. 2.76.*

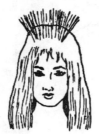

Fig. 2.76

Sides: 180 degree angle. *Fig. 2.77.*

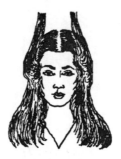

Fig. 2.77

Back: zero elevation. *Fig. 2.78.*

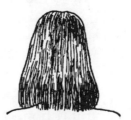

Fig. 2.78

LAYERED SECTIONS

Section thirteen corresponds to the top. *Fig. 2.79*.

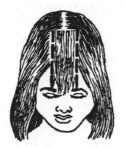

Fig. 2.79

Section fourteen, to the left side. *Fig. 2.80*.

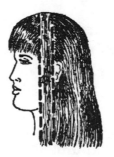

Fig. 2.80

Section fifteen, to the right side. *Fig. 2.81*.

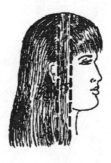

Fig. 2.81

CUTTING THE BOB

1. Cut a bob as explained on page 76 and angle the sides as explained in page 62.

Once this step is completed return to this page and proceed to cut the top and side layers as follows:

CUTTING THE LAYERS

Top: section thirteen

1. Re-establish ear-to-ear parting and pin the hair of the back out of your way to keep your parting clean.

2. Cut top-level checkpoint. See page 34 for details on how to cut this guide.

3. Stand next to the subject's left side.

4. Comb the top hair forward and make section thirteen, a two-inch wide section on top of the head from top-level checkpoint to the front.

5. Elevate section thirteen at a ninety-degree angle and center it using the nose as your guide.

6. Cut from top-level checkpoint to the front. Join those two points in a straight line. Do not cut into the checkpoint or the front outline, see that they drop uncut. Cut one-and-a-half to two inches at a time in small snips with the tips of the scissors. *Fig. 2.82.*

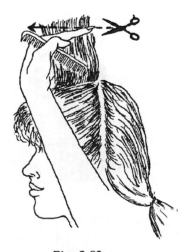

Fig. 2.82

Left Side: section fourteen

The sides have less hair. If the hair has been layered before, you'll only need one section on the sides. However, if you find that the hair is very thick and long, make two sections. Do the upper section first and cut it at top-level length, then lift the lower section and cut it level with the first.

1. Stand next to the subject's left side.

2. Elevate the section at a 180 degree angle in a horizontal direction and drop the perimeter.

3. Cut it at top-level length. *Fig. 2.83.*

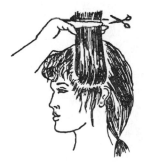

Fig. 2.83

If the length is very long you may need to over-extend the sides to avoid cutting the perimeter. *Fig. 2.84.* If you cut the perimeter while doing the layers, you will change its shape and length. See page 131 for details on how to measure the hair to make sure the perimeter does not reach the guide.

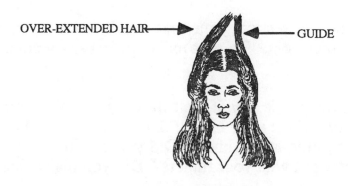

OVER-EXTENDED HAIR ⟶   ⟵ GUIDE

Fig. 2.84

Right Side: section fifteen

1. Stand next to the subject's right side.

2. Lift the section at a 180 degree angle and drop the perimeter.

3. Cut horizontally at top-level length. *Fig. 2.85.*

TOP GUIDE

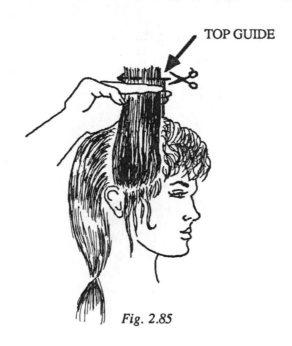

Fig. 2.85

4. Comb the hair of the sides to the back. If she is satisfied with the length of the layers go on to check the haircut. If she is not, trim the side outline and shorten the layers.

CHECKING

Once you have cut the last section, your next step is to check the haircut. If the sections are uneven, even them out. Do not make unnecessary cuts. Do not make new guides.

Ask yourself if you have made any of the following mistakes; they could be the reasons to uneven lengths of hair in your layers: Did you hold the hair at the correct angle? Did you follow the guide at all times? Did you part the hair correctly? Did you maintain the scissors straight with your fingers? Did you make clean partings?

1. Top: Stand behind the subject. Hold the hair at a ninety-degree angle and check the top in three horizontal sections. Start at top-level checkpoint and move towards the front. *Fig. 2.86.*

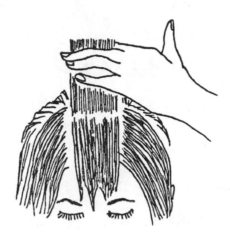

Fig. 2.86

2. Sides: Remain behind the subject. Re-adjust ear-to-ear parting. Elevate the sides at a 180 degree angle in a vertical direction and check that the line is straight with the top. *Fig. 2.87.*

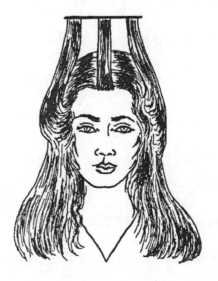

Fig.2.87

Now the haircut is completed.

REVIEW QUESTIONS

To ensure that you have learned the steps of the bob variation, answer the following questions. The page numbers next to the questions indicate where the answers can be found.

1. How would you explain what one-length is? p. 30

2. What facial faces look good with a bob variation? pp. 43-46

3. How would you part the back of the hair to cut a bob variation? p. 93

4. In what way is this haircut similar to the bob? p. 93

5. In what way is this haircut similar to the long-layered? p. 93

6. What are the guides used to cut the back? p. 94

7. At what degrees of elevation would you hold the hair to cut the back, the top and the sides? p. 94

8. How many layered sections are there? p. 95

9. Where would you start the haircut and where would you end it? pp. 96 and 98

10. What is the guide to the top length? p. 96

11. Why would you tie the hair of the back out of the way? p. 96

12. Is the hair of the sides cut in vertical or horizontal direction? p. 97

13. If the hair is very long, how would you make sure that you are not cutting the the outline? p. 97

14. What is the guide to the side layers? p. 98

15. Briefly explain how would you check the top and back of this haircut? p. 99

F. BI-LEVEL WITH BOBBED BACK

The bi-level with bobbed back is a combination of styles: The top and sides are cut in short layers as in a one-level; the back is one-length as in a bob.

With the one-level top, bounce and volume are accomplished. The sides, short and close to the head, open up the face, and the blunt cut in the back softens and frames the neck area. To change the looks of this style, the back may be pinned up for a sophisticated evening or a hot afternoon. *Fig. 2.88.*

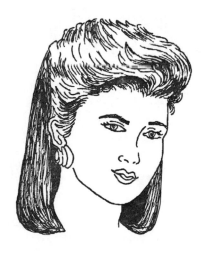

Fig. 2.88

PARTING THE HAIR

See illustrations of partings on Section D, page 77.

Top parting: center, from the crown to the forehead.

Side parting: from ear-to-ear.

Front parting: triangle, from one-third of the top to the temples.

Back parting: triangle, from the occipital bone to below the ears. Pin the upper
     section out of the way and smooth the rest of the hair down.

GUIDES

Back perimeter
Top of the nose   } OUTLINE
Temples
Eyebrows

Top-level checkpoint
Nose   } LAYERS
Top section
Sections and layers

ANGLES

Outline: zero elevation. *Fig. 2.89.*

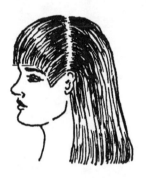
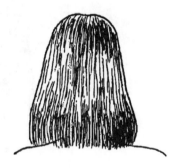

Fig. 2.89

Top and sides: ninety-degree angle. *Fig. 2.90.*

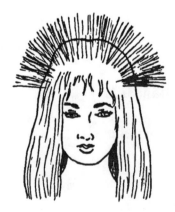
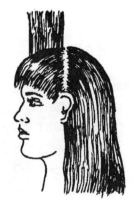

Fig. 2.90

LAYERED SECTIONS

Section seven corresponds to the top. *Fig. 2.91.*

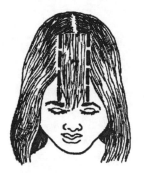

Fig. 2.91

Section eight, left side. *Fig. 2.92.*

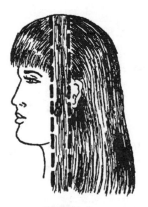

Fig. 2.92

Section nine, right side. *Fig. 2.93.*

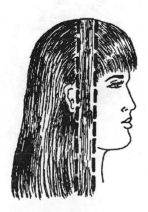

Fig. 2.93

CUTTING THE BACK

1. Cut a bob in the back. See Section D, page 82-85 for details on how to cut a bob back.

Once the back sections are completed return to this page and proceed to outline the front and the sides as follows:

TO OUTLINE THE FRONT

In this section of the outline act with care. As we mentioned before cowlicks and widow's peaks are common in the hairline.

a) From the Center to the Right Temple

1. Lift the subject's head straight.

2. Stand in front of the subject.

3. Re-adjust the triangle parting in the top.

4. Cut a center guide on top of the nose.

5. Cut from the top of the nose to below the temple. *Fig. 2.94.*

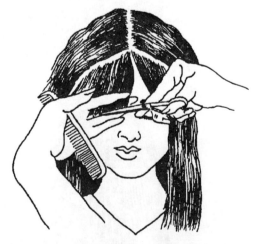

Fig. 2.94

Make sure the right side is even and get ready to cut the left side.

b) From the Center to the Left Temple

The left side of the front outline will be parted in two sections. This way you will always have your guide visible.

1. Cut section one and join it with the center guide. *Fig. 2.95.*

2. Cut section two from below the temple to section one and join them. Make sure you place your fingers in the same angle you had them on the other side *Fig. 2.96.*

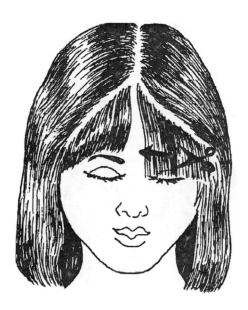

Fig. 2.95

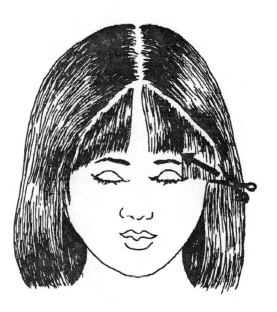

Fig. 2.96

3. Once the left side is finished stand back and observe. Do you have an even curvature? Is it too short, too long? If the hair is too long make a new guide in the center and start again. Adjustments should be made cutting one-quarter inch at a time. Remember that once the hair dries, it will be shorter.

4. Breath deeply and get ready to cut the sides.

a) Left Side

1. Re-establish ear-to-ear parting and pin up the hair of the back out of the way.

2. Stand next to the subject's left side.

3. Tilt the subject's head to the right side to have a clear view and a comfortable position to work.

4. Comb the hair down over the ear. *Fig. 2.97.*

5. Cut from the ear to the front the length agreed with the subject (top of the ear, mid-ear or below the ear). Do not cut above the hairline. *Fig. 2.97.*

6. Comb the hair toward the front. *Fig. 2.98.*

7. Drop the outline. Cut in a upward direction toward the temple and meet the frontal outline. *Fig. 2.98.*

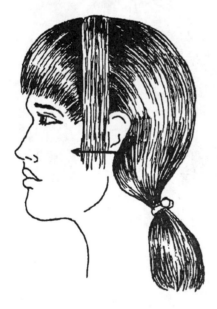

Fig. 2.97

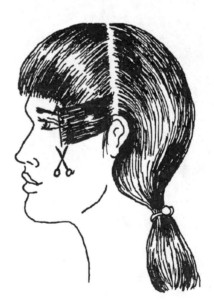

Fig. 2.98

Now the left side is finished. Make sure that the length is acceptable with the person and get ready to cut the right side.

b) Right Side

Once you are finished with the left side proceed to outline the right side using the same method.

1. Stand next to the subject's right side.

2. Re-adjust ear-to-ear parting.

3. Tilt the subject's head to the left side.

4. Comb the hair of the side over the ear. *Fig. 2.99.*

5. Cut from the front to the ear. *Fig. 2.99.*

6. Comb the hair towards the front. Fig. *2.100.*

7. Cut in a downward direction from below the temple to the cheek. *Fig. 2.100.*

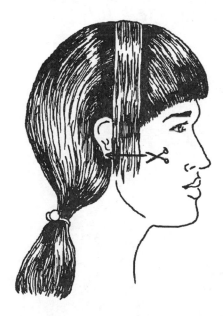

Fig. 2.99

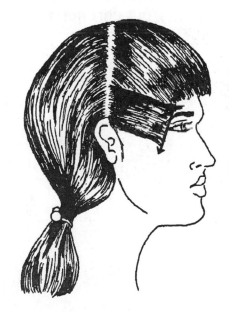

Fig. 2.100

Breath deeply; stand back and observe. You may use the bones of the ears as points of reference to make sure you have the same length on both sides.

Once the outline is completed we can start cutting layers on the top and side hair as follows:

CUTTING THE LAYERS

Top: section seven

1. Re-establish ear-to-ear parting and keep the hair of the back pinned out of your way.

2. Cut top-level checkpoint. See Section F, page 34 for details on how to cut this guide.

3. Stand next to the subject's left side.

4. Comb the hair of the top forward and make a two-inch wide section from top-level checkpoint to the front.

5. Elevate it at a ninety-degree angle and cut from top-level checkpoint to the front. Join those two points in a straight line. Do not cut into the checkpoint or the front perimeter, see that they drop uncut. *Fig. 2.101*.

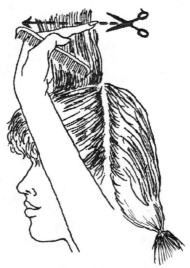

Fig. 2.101

Comb the top towards the back and make sure the length is acceptable. If it is too long, trim the top layer. Adjustments should be made cutting one-quarter inch at a time.

Left Side: section eight

1. Remain next to the subject's left side.

2. Comb section seven forward and make a center parting on the top.

3. Re-adjust ear-to-ear parting and keep the hair of the back pinned out of your way.

4. Hold section eight at a ninety-degree angle in vertical direction.

5. Cut from the perimeter to the top. Join section eight to section seven. *Fig. 2.102.*

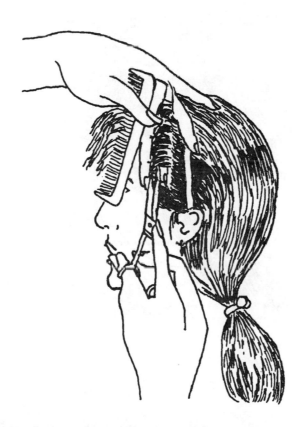

Fig. 2.102

Now the left side is completed. Comb the hair to the back and make sure that the length of the layers is acceptable. If it is not, trim the side outline and shorten the layers. Otherwise go on to the right side and cut it as follows:

Right Side: section nine

1. Stand behind the subject.

2. Elevate section nine at a ninety-degree angle. Make sure you are not pulling the section back towards you. If you do, it will be longer than section eight on the left side.

3. Cut from the perimeter to the top. Join section nine to section seven. *Fig. 2.103.*

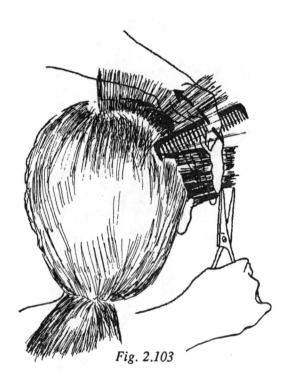

Fig. 2.103

CHECKING

Once you have cut the last section the next step is to check the haircut. If there are uneven sections, even them out. Do not make unnecessary cuts. Do not make new guides.

Ask yourself if you have made any of the following mistakes; they could be the reasons to uneven lengths of hair in your layers: Did you apply too much tension to some sections of hair? Did you follow the guide at all times? Did you make clean partings? Did you elevate the hair at the required angle?

Pin the hair of the back out of your way and stand behind the subject.

1. Top: Elevate the hair at a ninety-degree angle and check the top in three horizontal sections from the checkpoint to the front. *Fig. 2.104.*

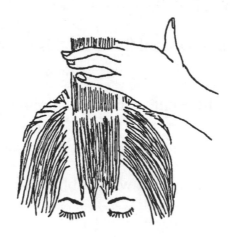

Fig. 2.104

2. Sides: Stand next to the subject to check the sides in horizontal sections at a ninety-degree angle. Start at the top and work your way down towards the hairline. *Fig. 2.105.*

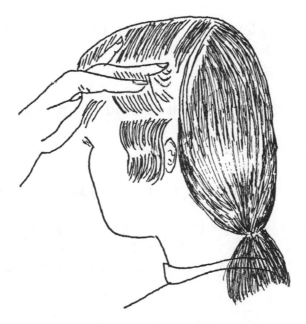

Fig. 2.105

Now the haircut is completed. Breath deeply and smile.

REVIEW QUESTIONS

To ensure that you have learned the steps to cut the bi-level with bobbed back, answer the following questions. The page numbers next to the questions indicate where the answers can be found.

1. If the face was long, how could you cut this haircut to help correct the features. pg. 44

2. How is this haircut different to the bob haircut? pg. 101

3. How is this haircut different to the one level haircut? pg. 101

4. How would you part a bi-level with bobbed back? pg. 101

5. List the guides to cut the back. pg. 102

6. List the guides to cut the top and sides. pg. 102

7. At what degree would you outline the hair? pg. 102

8. Would you elevate the hair to cut the back? pg. 102

9. At what degree of elevation would you layer the top and the sides? pg. 102

10. How many layered sections are there in this haircut? pg. 103

11. Explain the procedure to outline the sides. pp. 106-107

12. In what direction would you cut the sides? pg. 109

13. Where would you stand to layer the left side? the right side? pp. 109-110

14. Briefly explain how would you check this haircut. pg. 111

G. BI-LEVEL WITH LONG-LAYERED BACK

The bi-level combines two hairstyles: The one-level with short layers in the top and the sides, and the long-layered in the back.

This haircut is ideal for the person who enjoys the looks of short wavy hair around the face but does not want to lose their long hair in the back. By pinning up the hair this style offers different styling options, from the long look, to the short look. It is also a popular style among the men that prefer long hair with a tailored look. *Fig. 2.106.*

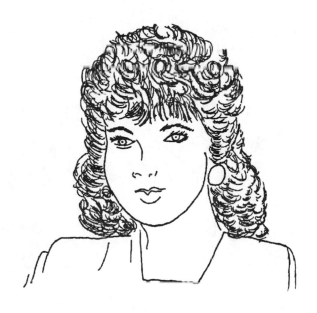

Fig. 2.106

PARTING THE HAIR

See illustrations of partings in Section A, page 51.

Top parting: center, from the crown to the forehead.

Side parting: from ear-to-ear.

Front parting: triangle, from one-third of the top to the temples.

Back parting: smooth it down with no partings.

GUIDES

Perimeter
Top of the nose   OUTLINE
Temples
Eyebrows

Crown-level checkpoint
Nose   LAYERS
Top section
Sections and layers

ANGLES

Top and sides: ninety-degree angle. *Fig. 2.107*.

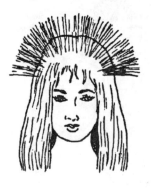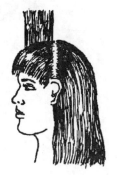

Fig. 2.107

Back: 180 degree angle. *Fig. 2.108*.

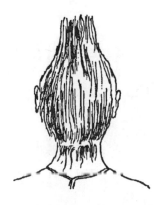

Fig. 2.108

LAYERED SECTIONS

Section one corresponds to the top. *Fig. 2.109*.

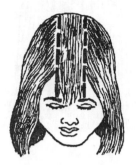

Fig. 2.109

Section two, left side. *Fig. 2.110*.

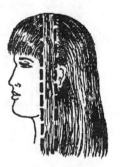

Fig. 2.110

Section three, right side. *Fig. 2.111*.

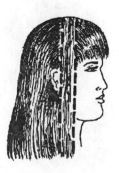

Fig. 2.111

Sections four and five, center of the back. *Fig. 2.112.*

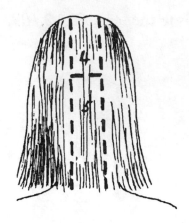

Fig. 2.112

Sections six and seven, left side of the back. *Fig. 2.113.*

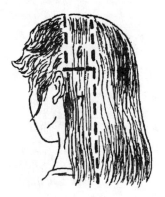

Fig. 2.113

Sections eight and nine, right side of the back. *Fig. 2.114.*

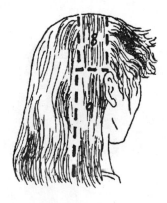

Fig. 2.114

OUTLINE

1. Outline the back, front and sides. See Section B, page 53 for details on how to outline the hair.

Once the outline is completed return to this page and proceed to cut the layers as follows:

CUTTING THE LAYERS

Top: section one

1. Stand next to the subject's left side.

2. Cut crown-level checkpoint. See Section F, page 34 for details on how to cut this guide.

3. Comb the top hair forward.

4. Make a two-inch wide section, from crown-level checkpoint to the front.

5. Elevate section one at a ninety-degree angle and align it with the subject's nose.

6. Cut from the checkpoint to the front. Join those two points in a straight line. Do not cut into the checkpoint or the front perimeter, see that they drop uncut. *Fig. 2.115.*

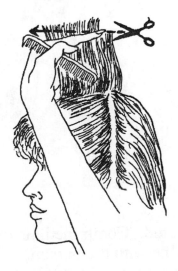

Fig. 2.115

Left Side: section two

1. Remain next to the subject's left side.

2. Make a center parting on the top.

3. Re-adjust ear-to-ear parting and pin the hair out of your way.

4. Cut section two from the perimeter to the top at a ninety-degree angle in a vertical direction. Use the perimeter as a guide to the length. *Fig. 2.116.*

5. Join section two to section one.

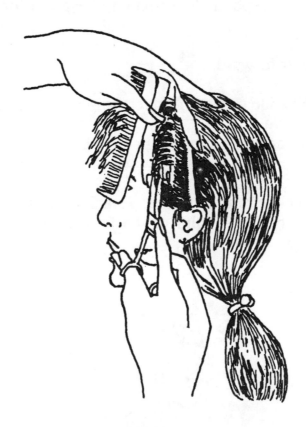

Fig. 2.116

Now the left side is completed. Comb the hair to the back and make sure that the length of the layers is acceptable with the person. If it is not, trim the side outline and shorten the layers. Otherwise cut the right side as follows:

Right Side: section three

1. Stand behind the subject's right shoulder.

2. Elevate section three at a ninety-degree angle.

3. Cut from the perimeter to the top in a vertical direction. Use the perimeter as a guide to the length. *Fig. 2.117.*

4. Join section three to section one.

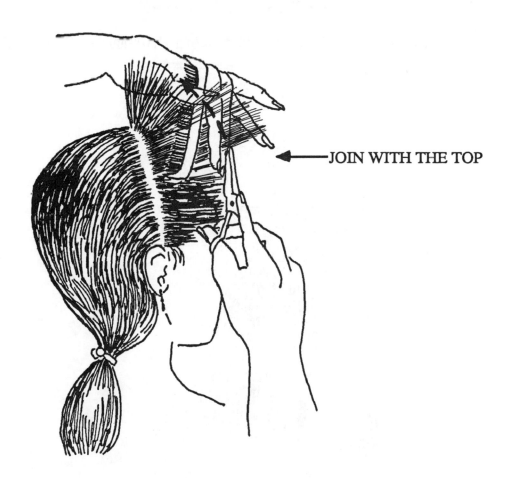

JOIN WITH THE TOP

Fig. 2.117

Now the sides are completed. Comb the hair and make sure both sides are equally long. Breath deeply and get ready to cut the back layers.

Back: sections four thru nine

When cutting the sections of the back under the occipital bone, be careful with the perimeter. If the hair is very long, you may need to over-extend the hair. If the hair does not reach the crown-level checkpoint when you lift it, just drop it and move to the next section. See Section H, page 131 for more details.

1. Stand behind the subject. Comb the hair of the back down.

2. Make section four, a rectangular in the middle of the back, from the crown to the occipital bone.

3. Elevate section four at a 180 degree angle. *Fig. 2.118*.

4. Cut section four at crown-level checkpoint in a horizontal direction. *Fig. 2.118*.

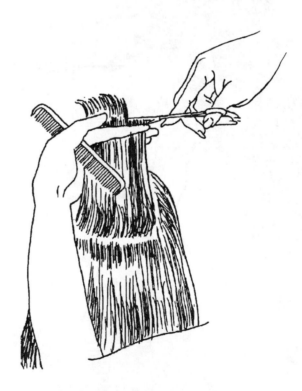

Fig. 2.118

5. Elevate section five at a 180 degree angle together with section four. Let the perimeter drop. Cut if there is hair extending over the crown-level checkpoint, otherwise drop the hair and continue to section six. *Fig. 2.119.*

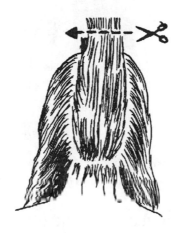

Fig 2.119

6. Make section six and include one-quarter inch of hair from section four as a guide to the length. *Fig. 2.120.*

7. Elevate and cut section six at a 180 degree angle. *Fig. 2.120.*

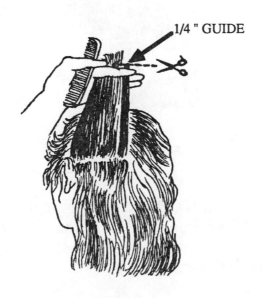

1/4 " GUIDE

Fig. 2.120

8. Elevate section seven at a 180 degree angle and cut it using section six as a guide. Cut if there is hair extending over section six. *Fig. 2.121.*

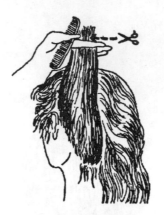

Fig. 2.'21

9. Elevate section eight on the right side of the back and cut it at a 180 degree angle. Use section four as a guide to the length. *Fig. 2.122.*

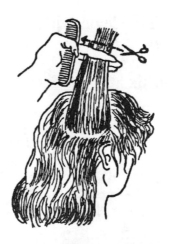

Fig. 2.122

10. Elevate section nine at a 180 degree angle together with section eight. Cut if there is hair extending beyond section eight. Otherwise drop the hair.

11. Breath deeply; comb the hair and observe.

12. The layers are now completed. Get ready to check the haircut.

CHECKING

Check the haircut and even out the sections with crooked lines. Do not make unnecessary cuts. Do not make new guides.

Ask yourself if you made any of the following mistakes; they could be the reasons to uneven lengths of hair in your sections: Did you apply too much tension to some sections of hair? Did you follow the guide of previous sections at all times? Did you part the hair correctly? Did you place your hand in the appropiate angle? Did you consistenly lift the hair at the required angle? Were some sections too big and others too small?

1. Crown: Stand behind the subject. Make a horizontal section at the crown. Elevate it at a 180 degree angle and even out if necessary. Ideally this section should be perfectly straight, if it is one-half inch longer on one side, it indicates that one side of the head has longer hair. If that's the case, start the haircut from the beginning. *Fig. 2.123*.

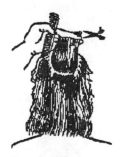

Fig. 2.123

2. Top: Stand behind the subject. Check the top in three horizontal sections from the crown to the front. Elevate the hair at a ninety-degree angle and if necessary even out the section. *Fig. 2.124*.

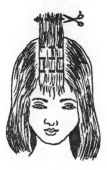

Fig. 2.124

3. Sides: Elevate the hair at a ninety-degree angle and check the sides in horizontal sections. *Fig. 2.125.*

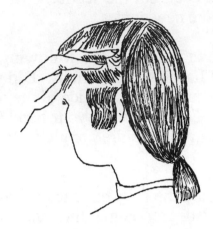

Fig. 2.125

4. Back: Elevate the hair at a 180 degree angle in vertical sections from the right side of the back to left side. *Fig. 2.126.*

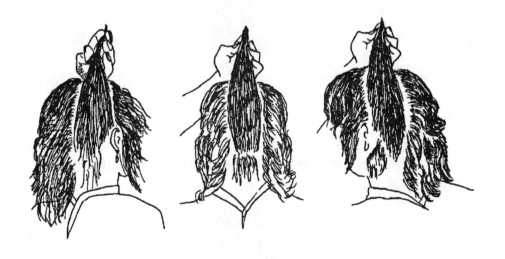

Fig. 2.126

Now the haircut is finished. Comb the hair and smile.

REVIEW QUESTIONS

To ensure that you have learned the steps to the bi-level with long-layered back, answer the following questions. The page numbers next to the questions indicate where the answers can be found.

1. In what way is this haircut similar to the one-level? p. 113

2. In what way is this haircut similar to the long-layered? p. 113

3. How would you part the hair? p. 113

4. At what angle would you cut the top and sides. p. 114

5. At what angle would you cut the back? p. 114

6. How many sections at the sides? p. 115

7. How many sections are there in the back? p. 116

8. In what direction would you cut the sides? p. 118

9. What are the guides to the top and side layers? pp. 117, 118

10. What would you do if the side layers are too long? p. 118

11. In what direction would you elevate and cut the hair of the back? p. 120

12. What would you do if the perimeter does not reach the top guide ? pp. 120, 131

13. What are the guides to the back layers? pp. 120-122

14. How can you make sure that you are not cutting the perimeter? p. 120

15. Briefly explain how would you check this haircut. pp. 123-124

H. LONG-LAYERED

This haircut is perfect to give fullness and bounce to wavy, curly and super-curly hair. It reduces hair bulk, and yet maintains the length long all over. It is the style that offers the most sexy, sophisticated looks. *Fig. 2.127.*

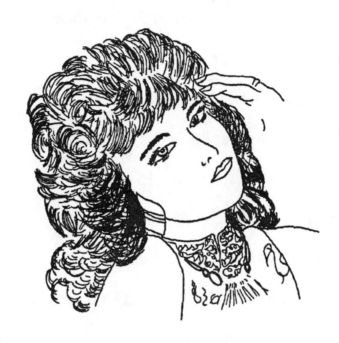

Fig. 2.127

PARTING THE HAIR

See illustrations of partings in Section A, page 51.

Top parting: center, from the crown to the forehead.

Side parting: from ear-to-ear.

Front parting: triangle, from one-third of the top to the temples.

Back: smooth it down with no partings.

GUIDES

Perimeter Top of the nose Temples Eyebrows	OUTLINE
Crown-level checkpoint Nose Top section Sections and layers	LAYERS

ANGLES

Top: ninety-degree angle. *Fig. 2.128.*

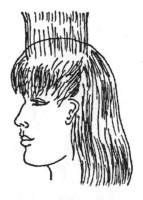

Fig. 2.128

Sides and back: 180 degree angle. *Fig. 2.129.*

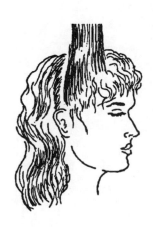 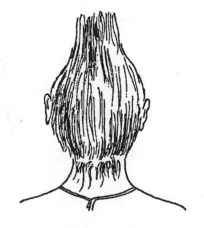

Fig. 2.129

LAYERED SECTIONS

Section one corresponds to the top. *Fig. 2.130*.

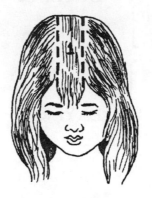

Fig. 2.130

Sections two and three, center of the back. *Fig. 2.131*.

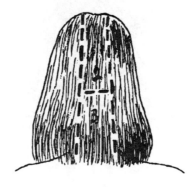

Fig. 2.131

Sections four and five, left side of the back. *Fig. 2.132*.

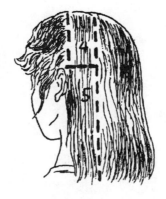

Fig. 2.132

Sections six and seven, right side of the back. *Fig. 2.133*.

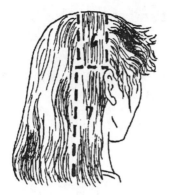

Fig. 2.133

Section eight, left side. *Fig. 2.134*.

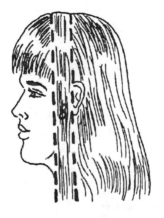

Fig. 2.134

Section nine, right side. *Fig. 2.135*.

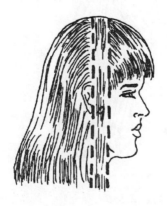

Fig. 2.135

OUTLINE

1. Outline the back, front and sides. See Section B, page 53 for details on how to outline the hair.

Once the outline is completed return to this page and proceed to cut the layers as follows:

CUTTING THE LAYERS

1. Stand behind the subject.

2. Cut crown-level checkpoint. See Section F, page 34 for details on how to cut this guide.

Top: section one

1. Make section one, a two-inch wide parting on the top of the head.

2. Elevate section one at a ninety-degree angle.

3. Cut from the checkpoint to the front. *Fig. 2.136.*

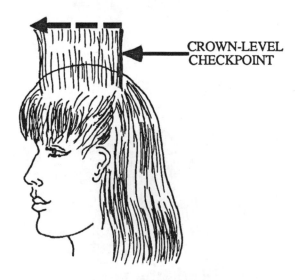

CROWN-LEVEL
CHECKPOINT

Fig. 2.136

Back: sections two thru seven

When the hair is elevated at a 180 degrees, the outline has to drop. (If you cut the outline while giving layers, you will change its length and shape.) In the beginning you may not be sure whether you are cutting the outline if the hair, being wet, sticks together as you elevate it. If you are afraid to miscalculate, cut the checkpoint, elevate a strand of hair from the hairline at 180 degree angle and hold it at the ends. Elevate the checkpoint at a ninety-degree angle and measure. This way you will know if the perimeter extends beyond the checkpoint.

If the hair is very long, you may find that the outline does not drop. In this case, you will need to over-extend the section to top-level checkpoint or further, to make sure that the perimeter will not be cut. With experience you will know by looking at the length of the hair, if it's necessary to over-extend the sections. *Fig. 2.137.*

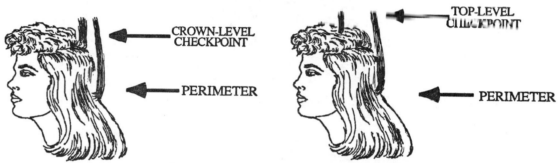

CROWN-LEVEL CHECKPOINT

PERIMETER

TOP-LEVEL CHECKPOINT

PERIMETER

MEASURE BY LIFTING THE CHECKPOINT AND THE PERIMETER

Fig. 2.137

1. Stand behind the subject.

2. Make section two, a two-inch wide parting from the crown to the occipital bone.

3. Elevate section two at a 180 degree angle and cut it at checkpoint-level length in a horizontal direction. *Fig. 2.138.*

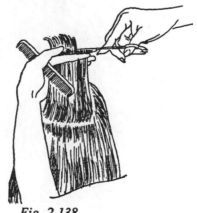

Fig. 2.138

4. Elevate section three at a 180 degree angle, allow the perimeter to drop. *Fig. 2.139.*

5. Cut the hair extending over the guide (section two). If the hair does not reach the guide just drop it and go on to the next section.

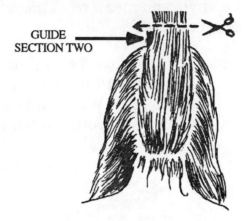

GUIDE
SECTION TWO

Fig. 2.139

6. Define section four in the left side of the back. Include one-quarter inch of section two as a guide to the length of section four.

7. Elevate and cut the hair at a 180 degree angle. *Fig. 2.140.*

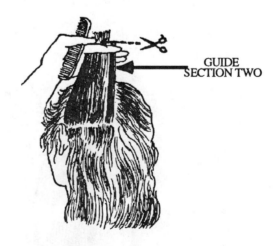

GUIDE
SECTION TWO

Fig. 2.140

8. Define section five from the occipital bone to the perimeter and elevate the section at a 180 degree angle.

9. Cut the hair extending over section four. *Fig. 2.141*.

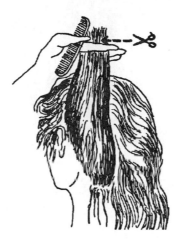

Fig. 2.141

10. Move to the right side of the back.

11. Lift and cut section six at a 180 degree angle. Include one-quarter inch of hair from section two as a guide to the length. *Fig. 2.142*.

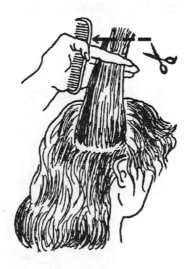

Fig. 2.142

133

2. Elevate section seven and repeat the same procedure. Use section six as a guide to the length. *Fig. 2.143*.

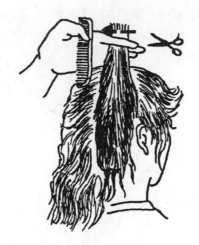

Fig. 2.143

Left Side: section eight

Usually the sides have less hair, especially if the hair has been layered before, so you'll only need one section at the sides. However, for very thick hair make two sections. If the hair is very long you may need to over-extend the hair to avoid cutting the outline. See page 97 for details.

1. Define section eight on the left side of the head.

2. Elevate it at a 180 degree angle, and cut it level with section one on the top of the head. *Fig. 2.144*.

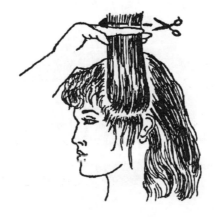

Fig. 2.44

Right Side: section nine

1. Repeat the procedure practiced on the left side to cut section nine. *Fig. 2.145.*

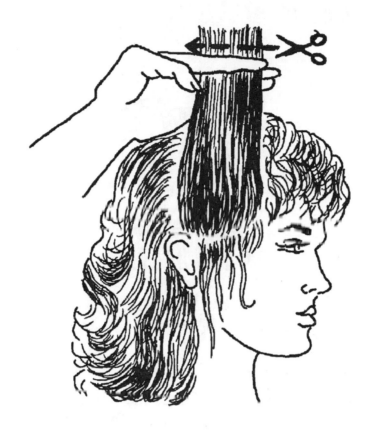

Fig. 2.145

2. Breath deeply and get ready to check the haircut.

CHECKING

When checking do not make unnecessary cuts or new guides. Even out the sections that are crooked or that have long wisps of hair.

Ask yourself if you made any of the following mistakes; they could be the reasons to uneven lengths of hair in your sections: Did you apply too much tension to some sections of hair? Did you follow the guide at all times? Did you part the hair correctly? Did some sections have more hair than others? Did you stretch the hair at the required angle?

1. Crown: Stand behind the subject. Elevate a horizontal section at the crown at a 180 degree angle and even it if necessary. Ideally it should be perfectly straight. If it is one-half inch or more longer on one side, it indicates that one side of the head has longer hair. If that is the case, start the haircut all over again. *Fig. 2.146*.

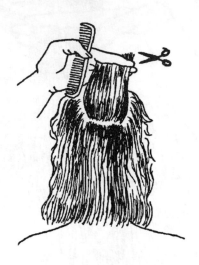

Fig. 2.146

2. Top: Stand behind the subject. Check the top at ninety-degree angle in three horizontal sections from the crown to the front. *Fig. 2.147*.

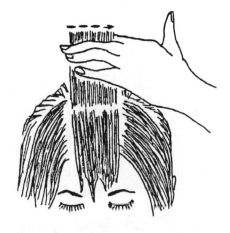

Fig. 2.147

3. Sides: Stand behind the subject. Elevate each side in vertical direction at a 180 degree angle. Make sure the line is straight with the top length. *Fig. 2.148.*

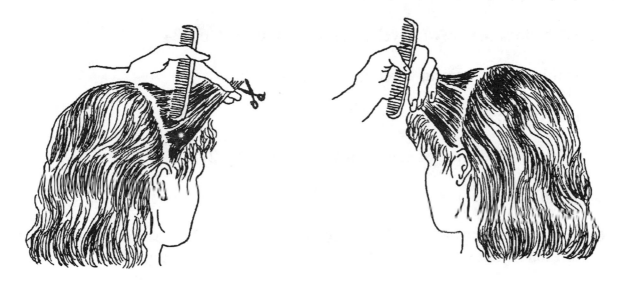

Fig. 2.148

4. Back: Starting at the right side of the back elevate the hair at a 180 degree angle in vertical sections. *Fig 2.149.*

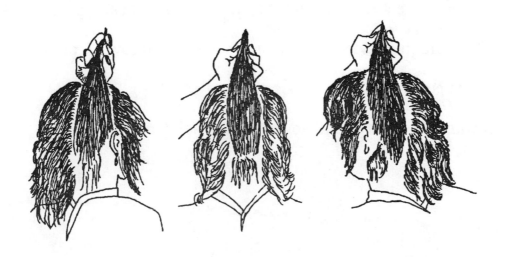

Fig. 2.149

REVIEW QUESTIONS

To ensure that you have learned the steps of the long-layered, answer the following questions. The page numbers next to the questions indicate where the answers can be found.

1. What does the crown-level checkpoint indicate? pg. 34

2. Is this a good haircut to reduce bulk? pg. 126

3. How is the hair parted? pg. 126

4. What is the degree of elevation at the top? pg. 127

5. What is the degree of elevation of the sides and the back? pg. 127

6. If you are not sure that the perimeter is dropping how would you be able to tell that it does not reach the crown-level checkpoint? pg. 131

7. Why, in some cases, would the hair need to be over-extended? pg. 131

8. In what direction are the layers cut? pg. 131

9. Why would you elevate the sections under the occipital bone together with the upper sections? pg. 132

10. Section two serves as a guide to what other sections? pp. 133-134

11. Which are the guides to sections three, five and seven? pp. 132-134

12. Which is the guide to sections nine and eight? pg. 135

13. In what direction would you check the hair? pp. 136-137

I. WEDGE

The wedge is an all time favorite. It is an easy-care, comfortable coif with a feminine touch. In the wedge we graduate the hair in reverse. The shortest point will be in the back perimeter and the longest at the crown. There are many variations of the wedge. Also the texture and density of the hair will change the looks of this style. *Fig. 2.150.*

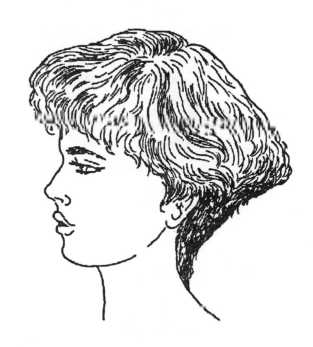

Fig. 2.150

PARTING THE HAIR

See illustrations of partings in Section A, page 51.

Top parting: center, from the crown to the forehead.

Side parting: from ear-to-ear.

Front parting: for bangs, triangle, from one-third of the top to the temples.

Back parting: V parting, from the top of the ears to the occipital bone. Pin the upper section out of the way, and smooth the rest of the hair down.

GUIDES

Perimeter
Top of the nose   } OUTLINE
Temples
Eyebrows

Sections and layers   } LAYERS

ANGLES

Back: zero elevation, forty-five-degree angle and 180 degree angle. *Fig. 2.51.*

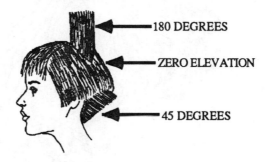

Fig. 2.151

Sides: forty-five-degree angle. *Fig. 2.152.*

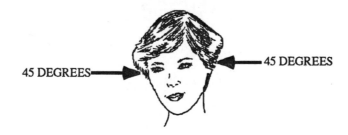

Fig. 2.152

Front: ninety-degree angle. *Fig. 2.153.*

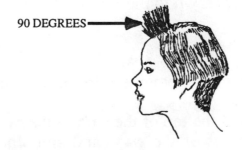

Fig. 2.153

LAYERED SECTIONS

The number of sections of the back may vary according to the size of the head, the width of the sections and the final look. Stop making sections when you reach the occipital bone. The sections should be approximately one-inch wide.

In our sample haircut we will have eight sections in the back.

Sections one thru eight, back. *Fig. 2.154.*

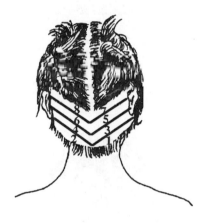

Fig. 2.154

Section nine, crown. *Fig. 2.155.*

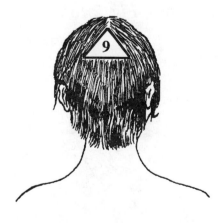

Fig. 2.155

Section ten, left side. *Fig. 2.156.*

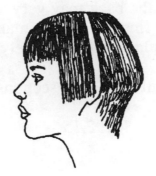

Fig. 2.156

Section eleven, right side. *Fig. 2.157.*

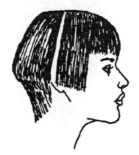

Fig. 2.157

Section twelve and thirteen, front. *Fig. 2.158.*

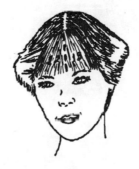

Fig. 2.158

OUTLINE

1. Outline the back, front and sides. See Section B, page 53 for details on how to outline the hair.

Once the outline is completed return to this page and proceed to cut the layers as follows:

CUTTING THE LAYERS

Back: sections one thru eight

1. Make the first section and pin up the rest of the hair out of the way.

2. Elevate the perimeter and section one at a forty-five-degree angle. *Fig. 2.159.*

3. Cut the section using the perimeter as a guide to the length. Do not cut into the perimeter, see that it drops uncut.

4. Cut horizontally from the right to the center in a downward direction to follow the contour of the head.

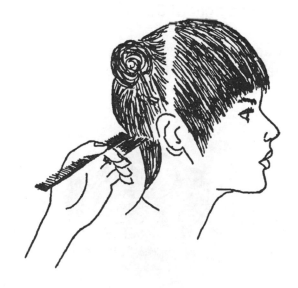

Fig. 2.159

5. Define section two.

6. Elevate it with the perimeter at a forty-five-degree angle. *Fig. 2.160*.

7. Cut from the center to the left in an upward direction. Use the perimeter and section one as your guides to length. In this way you'll be overlapping the sections for a blended effect in the layers.

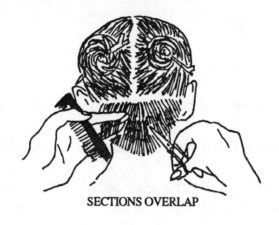

SECTIONS OVERLAP

Fig. 2.160

8. Bring down section three and four.

9. Pin up the rest of the hair out of the way.

10. Elevate section one and three at a forty-five-degree angle. Use section one as your guide. Make sure you do not cut section one, but that it drops uncut. *Fig. 2.161*.

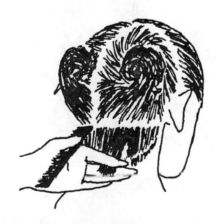

Fig. 2.161

11. Repeat the same steps with section four.

12. Continue the same procedure with each section until you reach the occipital bone.

Crown: section nine

1. Make section nine, a triangle at the crown.

2. Lift the hair at a 180 degree angle. If there is a point cut it straight and drop the hair. This procedure will keep the hair from flipping up at the ends. *Fig. 2.162.*

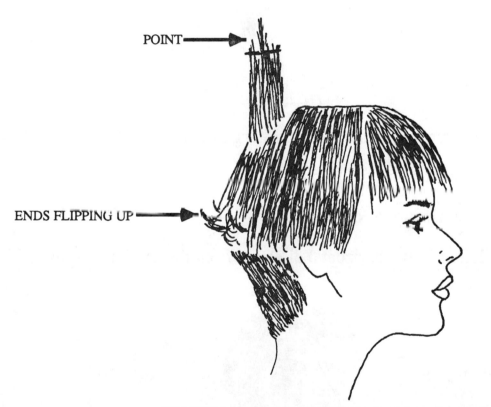

CUT THE POINT TO KEEP THE HAIR FROM FLIPPING UP.

Fig. 2.162

Now the back is completed. Breath deeply and get ready to cut section ten on the left side of the subject.

Section Ten: left side

If the hair of the sides is very thick, you may need to part it in half-horizontals. Cut the first layer at a forty-five-degree angle using the perimeter as your guide. Cut the second layer at a forty-five-degree angle using the length of the first layer as your guide. *Fig. 2.163*.

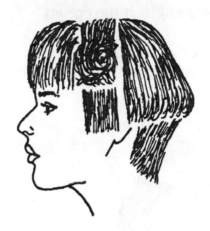

Fig. 2.163

1. Elevate the left side at a forty-five-degree angle in a horizontal direction. *Fig. 2.164*.

2. Use the perimeter as a guide to the length.

3. Allow the perimeter to drop.

4. Cut the left side in a horizontal direction from the ear to the front.

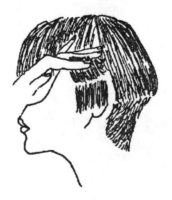

Fig. 2.164

Rigth Side: section eleven

1. Repeat the same procedure practiced on the left side to cut the right side.

You have now completed the sides. Breath deeply and get ready to cut the front as follows:

Front: sections twelve and thirteen

1. Elevate the left side at a ninety-degree angle.

2. Drop the perimeter.

3. Cut the ends in a horizontal direction from the temple to the center. *Fig. 2.165.*

4. Repeat the procedure with the right side of the front. Cut the ends from the center to the temple. Now the front is slightly layered. For a more layered look see Chapter III, page 153.

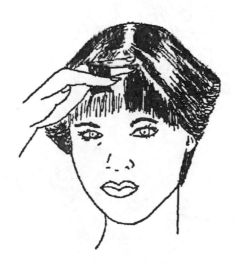

Fig. 2.165

You have now completed the front. Breath deeply, comb the hair, observe and get ready to check the haircut.

CHECKING

Ask yourself if you made any of the following mistakes; they could be the reasons to uneven lengths of hair in your sections: Did you apply too much tension to some sections of hair? Did you follow the guide at all times? Did you part the hair correctly? Did some sections have more hair than others? Did you place your hand in the appropiate angle? Did you stretch the hair at the required angle? Did you cut into the guide?

When checking do not make unnecessary cuts or new guides, simply even out the sections that are slightly crooked.

1. Back: Elevate the back at forty-five-degrees in vertical sections. Move from the center to the right and from the center to the left. The hair must be increasingly longer from the hairline to the occipital bone. *Fig. 2.166.*

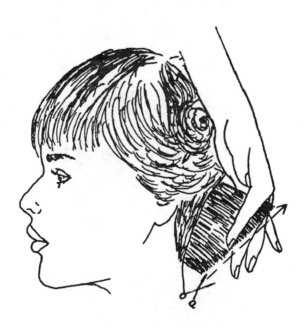

Fig 2.166

2. Sides: Elevate the hair at forty-five-degrees from the ear to the front in vertical sections. The hair must be increasingly longer from the perimeter to above the ears. *Fig. 2.167.*

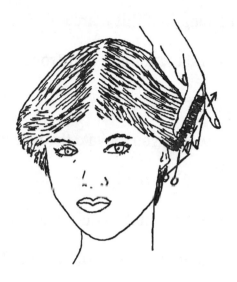

Fig. 2.167

3. Front: Check in vertical sections at a forty-five-degree angle. Move from the center to the right side and from the center to the left side. *Fig. 2.168.*

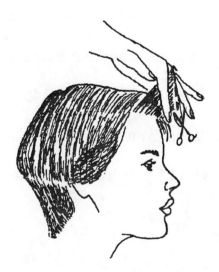

Fig. 2.168

REVIEW QUESTIONS

To ensure that you have learned the steps of the wedge, answer the following questions. The page numbers next to the questions indicate where the answers can be found.

1. How short should the length of this haircut be? p. 53

2. Where is the shortest and the longest hair from the crown? p. 139

3. How should the wedge be parted? p. 139

4. At what degree-angle would you elevate the hair to cut a wedge? p. 140

5. What are the guides to cut the outline? p. 140

6. How many sections are there in the back, sides and front? pp. 141-142

7 Which is the initial guide to the length of the back? p. 143

8. Are the layers cut in a vertical or horizontal direction? p. 143

9. List other guides to the sections of the back? p. 144

10. Why is there a section on the crown? p. 145

11. At what point should you stop making layers in the back? p. 145

12. If the hair is thick how would you part the sides? p. 146

13. How would you layer the sides and the front? pp. 146, 147

14. How would you check the back? pp. 148-149

15. How would you check the front and sides? p. 149

16. To check the hair, would you hold the hair in a horizontal or a vertical direction? p. 149

Chapter III

MORE TECHNIQUE

Once you have practiced the basic haircuts explained in Chapter II, you will be prepared to learn techniques to give accent to the haircuts. With these easy techniques you can emphasize movement of the hair in one direction, provide lift to the top, frame the face, provide extra layers to the front, and give character to the back.

Read through the different techniques and practice them later.

How to Cut Wisps of Hair

A few strands of hair in the front or in the sideburn area give softness and are flattering to the face.

Wisps are light and the hair will tend to curl more than bangs would. Also as we know, the hair around the hairline has cowlicks that will tend to curl it up or to the sides. For these reasons, it is best to cut the guide below the eyebrows, and to cut the wisps without stretching the hair with tension. Cut the wisps semi-dry to see in which direction the hair tends to move. To make wisps on the forehead follow the steps below:

1. Ask the person how much hair she likes to have covering her forehead. The more hair you take, the more the wisps will resemble bangs.

2. Cut a strand in the middle of the forehead and make sure this length is acceptable. This will be your guide.

3. Hold all the hair selected in the center of the forehead.

4. Slide your fingers to the ends of the guide, when the guide snaps released, cut above the fingers. *Fig. 3.1*.

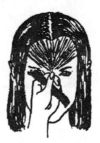

Fig. 3.1

To give sideburn wisps bring hairline hair down and cut no shorter than the length of the ear. *Fig. 3.2*. Comb the hair towards the cheek and shape it. *Fig. 3.3*.

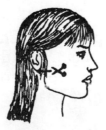

Fig. 3.2

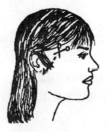

Fig. 3.3

How to Layer Bangs

Bangs can sometimes have a very heavy and thick appearance. To make them lighter and give them a layered look, proceed as follows:

1. Make a triangle parting from one-third of the top to the temples.

2. Elevate the section at a ninety-degree angle in a vertical direction. *Fig. 3.4.*

3. Allow the outline to drop.

4. Cut the ends of the hair at a ninety-degree angle. *Fig. 3.5.*

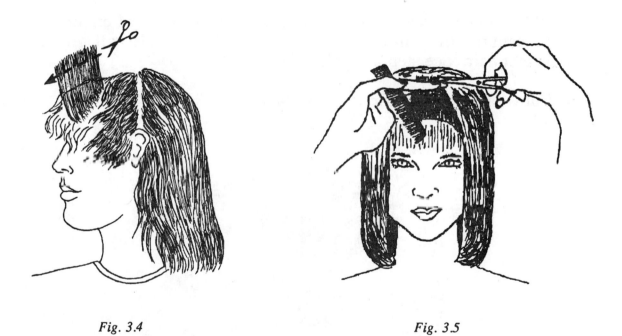

Fig. 3.4   *Fig. 3.5*

5. Elevate the bangs again; this time in a horizontal position and trim any uneven ends.

How to Spike the Hair of the Top

The hair can be layered or it can be one-length. To spike the top proceed as follows:

(To give less dramatic spikes, use the top-level checkpoint instead.)

1. Make triangle parting from crown-level checkpoint to the temples.

2. Make crown-level checkpoint.

3. Elevate the section at a ninety-degree angle.

4. Cut the hair, from crown-level checkpoint to the front, about two inches long or as short as you can without making the hair stick up. See step 1, fig. 3.6.

5. With thinning shears, cut the same section an inch away from the scalp. This procedure will remove weight and the shorter ends will give lift to the longer hair. See step 2, fig. 3.6.

6. Cut with thinning shears only two times.

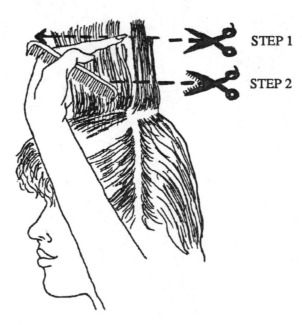

Fig. 3.6

7. To keep the spikes sticking up, style the hair with mousse, gel, hair spray or setting lotion.

How to Cut the Top for Forward Motion

If you want the top to move forward, the crown hair needs to be longer than the front hair. Cut as follows:

1. Cut the outline.

2. Cut crown-level checkpoint if the hair is layered, or top-level checkpoint if the haircut has a bobbed back.

3. Make a triangular parting from the checkpoint to the front.

4. Elevate the hair at a ninety-degree angle and place your fingers downward to give less length to the front. *Fig. 3.7.*

5. Cut from checkpoint to the front. Make sure the outline drops uncut.

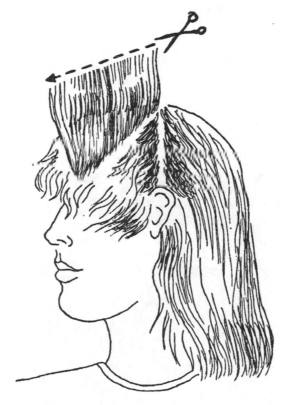

Fig. 3.7

6. If the hair is too thick in front, elevate one-third of the front hair and cut it twice with thinning shears. Keep a distance of two inches from the scalp. Remember, do not thin out hairline hair. *Fig. 3.7.*

How to Cut the Top for Backward Motion

If you want the top hair to move backward, you need the front hair to be longer than the crown hair. Cut it as follows:

1. Cut the outline.

2. Cut crown-level checkpoint if the hair is layered, or top-level checkpoint if the haircut has a bobbed back.

3. Make a triangular parting from the checkpoint to the front.

4. Elevate the hair at a ninety-degree angle and place your fingers in an upward direction to give length to the front.

5. Cut from the checkpoint to the front. *Fig. 3.8.*

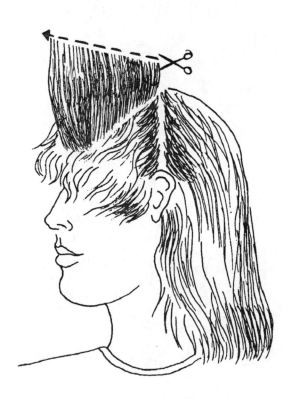

Fig. 3.8

How to Cut Ducktails

To make the ducktails you need the hair of the center back to be the shortest point. The hair has to increase in length as it gets closer to the back of the ears.

1. Shape the outline.

2. Make a quarter-inch section in the center and cut it to make a guide.

3. Make vertical sections moving from the center to the back of the ears.

4. Hold the hair towards the center and cut the sections at a forty-five-degree angle. *Fig. 3.9.*

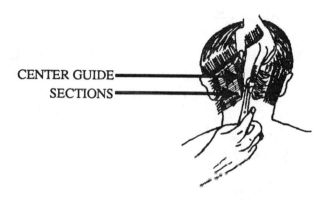

CENTER GUIDE

SECTIONS

Fig. 3.9

If you have completed a one-level haircut and the subject wants the look of ducktails, gather the hair of the back in the center and elevate it at a ninety-degree angle. Cut from the perimeter to the occipital bone. *Fig. 3.10.*

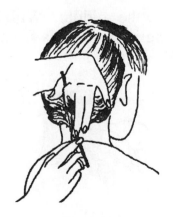

Fig. 3.10

157

How to Blow-Style the Hair

To blow-dry the hair after the haircut is finished make sure the hair is not wet, but evenly damp   If it is wet, towel dry it first. Remember that on page nineteen we discussed how the hair stretches when it is wet, and how it gets shorter when it is dry. When you apply heat to wet stretched hair it will contract and cause breakage.

Use the appropiate brush for the length and type of hair.   There are many kinds to choose. There are half-round brushes in different sizes good for rolling motions. A brush that allows the air to pass through for quick drying, is the vent brush. Radial brushes are great to style the bob and bob variations. The small radial brushes are useful in one-level haircuts, bi-levels and layered tops and sides. With these brushes you can give direction and volumen to the hair. Keep in mind that more people today want a natural finish. Also a style which doesn't require forcing the hair in place by overheating it is much preferable and less damaging to the hair.

To protect the hair from damage use a low-alcohol blow-drying lotion. Black hair will do fine with a light conditioner such as Fermodyl worked in damp hair. After the hair is retouched with the curling iron, a low-alcohol hair spray will maintain the final touches. You can apply mousse to keep the hair in place without the hard finish of a hair spray.   Aim the blow-drier upwards from the roots to the ends, or use a diffuser to give a smoother finish with no fly-away hair.

Blow-dry the roots first to give the style its shape, then do the ends. Keep the blow-dryer at least six inches away to avoid burning the scalp or the hair, and watch out for the ears, they often get burned. Divide the hair in sections to keep the drying organized. Do not roll thick sections of hair, instead roll sections approximately two inches wide if the hair is short. If the hair is long your sections will need to be smaller. If you take small sections you will do a better job and will finish faster.

For quick blow-drying try the following technique:

1. Part the hair of the back in the middle. With a radial brush dry the base of the hair. Then start drying it in sections from the center to behind the ears on either side of the back. *Fig. 3.11*.

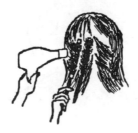

Fig. 3.11

3. Next, blow-dry the sides. *Fig. 3.12*

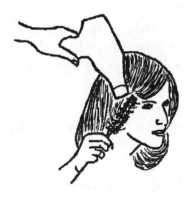

Fig. 3.12

4. Finally, do the top following the natural direction of the hair. *Fig. 3.13*.

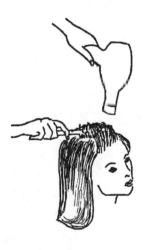

Fig. 3.13

For a sleeker look, set the waves with the curling iron. Roll the hair of the back in small sections with the curling iron. To make sure that you don't burn the hair, place a finger on the hair that has been rolled, count to ten and release the hair. If you feel your finger getting too hot, release the hair immediately. Let the curl cool before brushing.

For extra volume, apply mousse to towel dried hair, tilt the head down and dry it with a vent brush or fingers. Throw the hair back and arrange it with a hair pick. Apply hair spray for a lasting set.

For more lift on the top and sides apply gel to the roots of the hair and dry them with a vent brush by lifting the hair straight. When the hair has been completely blow-styled lift the hair with a hair pick and apply a spritz of hair spray to the roots to maintain the lift.

For contour, blow-dry the hair with a radial brush appropiate to the length of the hair.

For a more natural casual look, blow-dry the hair between your fingers holding it straight out to give it lift.

For more curls try scrunch drying. Squeeze the hair in a fist and allow the air to circulate through your fingers. When each section is dry, switch the dryer to a cool setting to fix the curl. Scrunch drying gives good results in combination with the diffuser. *Fig. 3.14*

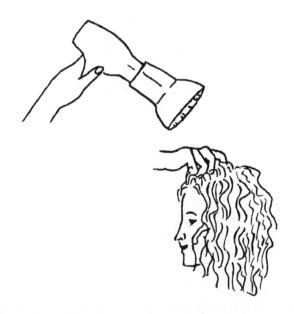

Fig. 3.14

Chapter IV

ANALIZING THE HAIR

To analize the hair means to examine it and determine whether it is damaged or healthy. The analysis is accomplished by observing and feeling the hair.

When analizing the hair reflect on the following questions. Is it chemically processed? Are the ends dry and split? Is the hair shaft faded or lacking shine? Is the scalp irritated?

Once the scalp and the hair are examined you can run your fingers down the length of a strand of hair stretching it. If the hair doesn't break but shows elasticity and turns into a new curl when released, the hair shaft is healthy and a trim can take care of damaged ends. If only half of the hair shaft turns into a new curl and breaks easily, you will know that the hair lacks elasticity because it is structurally weak or severely damaged. In this case, you will have to determine where and how this damage originated.

As you cut the hair, it is a good practice to indicate which areas are damaged. Find out the reasons to this damage and discuss with the person what should be done to correct it. You may ask the person questions about her activities, sports, hobbies and health.

How does she style and take care of her hair? What kind of brush is she using? Is she damaging her hair with chemicals, sun, hot rollers, etc.? Is the hair brushed when wet rather than properly combed. Is it ever conditioned? Is the hair frequently washed with a pH balanced shampoo suited to the needs of the hair--normal, oily, dry or chemically treated--?

The answers to these questions will give you clues to why the hair is damaged. In turn, you will be able to educate the individual recommending the changes, products and treatments, such as deep conditioning treatments, that will help avoid damage, and make the hair look better.

Another question you need to discuss with the person is how should the hair be washed. Point out that stimulating the blood flow is important to maintain healthy hair. Explain how easily this can be accomplished by massaging the scalp during each shampoo with the tips of the fingers, not with the nails.

Dry hair should be washed frequently with shampoo for dry hair and well conditioned for best results. Black hair should be frequently washed to restore the moisture balance that it needs or it will be more prone to damage. Keratin conditioners, low ph shampoos and conditioners, deep conditioners, and low-alcohol products are recommended for these types of hair. Emphasize that it is important to rinse thoroughly after shampooing and conditioning the hair. According to the needs of the hair, the types of shampoos and conditoner should be changed to compensate for the harmful effects of the weather, activities or environmental conditions.

It is a good practice to brush the hair from nape to top with the head down before retiring for the night. This will stimulate circulation increasing the blood flow to the roots of the hair. It will also help maintain the hair and the scalp healthy and dandruff free; and it will brush the dust out of the hair while distributing the oils from the scalp to the dry ends, serving as a natural conditioner. This procedure should be practiced regularly with a good brush that will not brake the hair or scratch the scalp. Also, brushing the hair before shampooing will result in cleaner hair. Make sure to analize the hair before engaging or recommending this practice. If the hair lacks elasticity it may cause breakage. If the hair is healthy brushing it twenty to thirty times is sufficient.

Explain the importance of regular trims to keep the hair healthy and shaped. Point out that in those areas where more length is desired, this can be achieved by cutting only where it is necessary or by trimming less than the hair growth during the period in between trims.

Happy haircuts!

APPENDIX

RESOURCES

To obtain quality scissors check the Yellow Pages for major beauty supplies in your area, or write or call the names below for distribution centers. Mention this book in your letters, subscriptions and inquiries.

F.W. Engels, Inc.
Dept. S - 55 West Hills Rd.
Huntington Station, New York 11746

Diana Products, Inc.   (Catalog available)
330 Fairfield Road
Fairfield, NJ 07006-1998

Fromm Industries   (Quality Japanese-Korean scissors)
For information call Toll Free: 1-800-323-4252

Conair   (Quality Japanese scissors)
Professional Products Division
Conair Corporation
Stamford, CT 06904

Tokosha Co. Ltd.   (Quality Japanese scissors)
4055 Wilshire Bl
Los Angeles, CA 90010

For information call Toll Free: 1-800-228-9739

To sharpen your fine shears contact:

Scott Roskam's   (For infomation call collect (213) 378-3555. Also will pick up at salons.)
Custom Sharpening by Hand
P.O. Box 3754
Torrance, Ca 90510

Publications:

USA

AHBIA News
111 E. Wacker Dr.
Suite 600
Chicago IL 60601

Quarterly. Covers Black issues in the cosmetology industry, news about products and trends.

American Salon
7500 Old Oak Boulevard
Cleveland, Ohio 44130

Monthly.   Salon news, hairstyles, products.

Modern Salon
400 Knightsbridge Pkwy
Lincolnshire, IL 60069

Monthly.   News, articles, tips, products.

Canada

Canadian Hairdresser
5200 Dixie Rd. Suite 204
Mississauga, Ont L4W 1E4

Text in English. Bi-monthly. News about products. Salon deco. Competition announcements.

France

La Coiffeur de France
1-3 place de la Bourse
75008 Paris

Text in French. Monthly. News, products, hairstyles. Has quarterly supplement with news and hair techniques.

La Coiffure De Paris
38 Rue Jean-Mermoz
75008 Paris

Monthly.   Text in French.   Hairstyling trends and products.   Write to agent in the USA: Modern Salon A Vance Publication P.O. Box 400, Prairie View IL 60069

Peluquerias
229 Rue Saint-Honoré
75001 Paris

Monthly. Text in French. Hairstyles and techniques.

Mariages
38 Rue Jean-Mermoz
75008 Paris

Text in French. Quarterly. Wedding hairdressing techniques step-by-step.

Hong Kong

Hair International
15th Floor, Lockhart Centre
301-307A Lockhart Road

Text in Chinese and English. Quaterly. Features hair care and Avant-Garde trends, techniques and products.

United Kingdom

Hair
Oakfield House
Perrymount Road
Haywards Heath, West Sussex RH 16 3 DH

Quaterly.   Hairstyle selection guide with 250 different styles.

Haidressers Journal International
Quadrant House The Quadrant
Sutton Surrey SM2 5AS

Weekly. Hairdesign competition news. Interviews. Points on hair color, hairstyles. Classified.

Bibliography

Blanchard, Leslie. *Foolproof Guide to Beautiful Hair*. New York: Dalton, 1988.

Borston Maurice, and Bloomfield Norma. *How to Blow Style*. Nottinhorn: Permaid Publications, 1975.

Chadwick, John. *The Chadwick System: Discovering the Perfect Hairstyle for You*. New York: Volkmann, 1982.

Charles, Ann. *The History of Hair*. New York: Bonanza, 1970.

Colletti, Anthony B. *Cosmetology The Keystone Guide to Beauty Culture*. Seventh Edition. New York. Keystone Publications, 1981.

Fodera, Sal. *Family Guide to Haircutting and Styling*. Drake, 1977.

Fine, Linda Sue. *The Complete Book of Hair Care, Hairstyling and Hairstylists*. New York: Arco Publishing, 1980.

Hofler, Robert. *Wild Style*. New York: Simon & Schuster, 1985.

Home Haircutting Made Easy /by the editors of Consumer Guide. New York: Bukman House: Distibuted by Crown Publishers, 1980.

Kenneth's Complete Book on Hair. Garden City. New York: Doubleday, 1972.

Lisa Layne. *The Simple Guide to Home Haircutting*. New York: Pinnacle Books, 1982.

Michael, George. *George Michael's Secrets for Beautiful Hair*. George Michael and Lindsay. Garden City. New York: 1981.

Morrison, Maggie. *Glamour Guide to Hair*. New York: Fawcett Columbine, 1986.

Ohnstad, Bob. *Scissors and Comb Haircutting*: Minneapolis, Minn.: You can Publish, 1985.

Roppatte, Vincent. *The Looks Men Love*. New York: St. Martin's Press, 1985.

The AMA Book of Skin and Hair Care. ed. Linda Allen Schoen. Philadelphia and New York: J.B. Lippincott, 1986.

Glossary

blunt cut- hair cut straight accross.
circulation- passage of blood through the body.
coarse hair- hair fiber large in diameter.
coif- hairstyle.
concave- curved inward.
conditioner- product to improve the appearance and feel of the hair.
contract- shrink.
convex- surface that curves outward, opposed to concave.
cowlick- tuft of hair forming a spiral turn.
degree- unit of measure for angles.
density- thickness.
dexterity- skill.
diffusser- hair-blower attachment to spread the air and heat.
ducktail- style for the back of the head. The hair meets in the center.
dry hair- hair devoid of enough natural oils.
elevate- lift.
extend- stretch out.
fine hair- term to identify the texture of the hair fiber small in diameter.
graduations- lengths.
hairline- edge of the scalp where the hair begins.
horizontal- parallel to the ground. From left to right as opposed to up and down.
increasingly- to become greater in size.
limp- lacking firmness or strength.
methodical- orderly, systematical.
medium hair- term to identify the texture of the hair fiber between fine and coarse.
nozzle- hair-blower attachment that directs the hair to one spot.
perimeter- outer boundary.
pH- the symbol for hydrogen ion concentration. pH scale expresses the degree of acidity or alkalinity in numbers from 0 to 14.
precision haircutting- hair cut with exactness, where the lengths are measured and even.
profile- side view of the face.
progressive- successive steps.
radial brush- round brush.
scrunch drying- technique to curl the hair with the hand while blow-drying it.
spikes- hair standing up.
sleeker- smooth, neat.
symmetrical- similar form on either side of the head.
tapered- gradually decreasing hair length.
texture- quality of the hair, coarse, medium or fine.
variables- changeable.
vent brush- brush designed to allow the hair to run thru to speed dry.
vertical- perpendicular to the ground. Moving up and down as opposed to left and rigth.
widow's peak- V shaped hairline at the middle of the forehead.

INDEX

A

B

C

D

E

HAIRCUTTING BASICS VIDEOTAPE

45 minutes of fun learning haircutting technique with music, live models and in full color in the privacy of your own home

Now you can feel confident when you cut hair. Practice at home, gain speed and make **more money!**

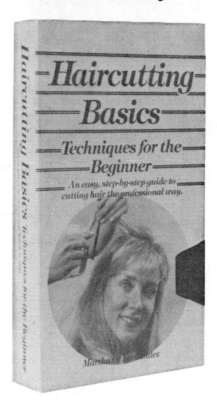

"Both tape and manual go together as back and forth reference, and for speed in a beauty salon, studying tape and manual has meant more money too."

Richard G. Lee
Cosmetologist
Miami, Fl

Haircutting Basics Videotape is to be used in conjunction with your book. Complete your learning program with the videotape that <u>shows in action</u> the step-by-step technique explained in the book.

Videotape covers Chapter II, Technique: How to cut a one-level, bob, bob variation, bi-level with bobbed back, bi-level with long-layered back, long-layered and wedge.

To order, fill out coupon in the next page.

ORDER FORM

NO RISK -- MONEY BACK GUARANTEE IF YOU'RE NOT SATISFIED!

		Quantity	Total
Haircutting Basics book (paperback)	@ **$16.95**	_____	_____
Haircutting Basics book (hardback)	@ **$24.95**	_____	_____
Haircutting Basics videotape	@ **$39.95**	_____	_____
Corte de Pelo Tecnica Basica (Spanish video)	@ **$39.95**	_____	_____
Paperback and videotape at package price	@ **$49.95**	_____	_____
Hardback and videotape at package price	@ **$56.95**	_____	_____

Sub-Total _____

Shipping: $1.00 for the first item and $0.50 for each additional item. _____

For videos, please circle. VHS   Beta   No COD orders please   **Total** _____

Name _____   Phone ( )_____

Address _____

City/State/Zip _____

_____ My check/money order is enclosed   _____ Bill my **American Express**   Card

Acct. # [ ][ ][ ][ ][ ][ ][ ][ ][ ][ ][ ][ ][ ][ ]   Expires _____   Signature _____

Mail to: Good Life Products, Inc., P. O. Box 5122, Hialeah, FL 33014-1122

ORDER FORM

NO RISK -- MONEY BACK GUARANTEE IF YOU'RE NOT SATISFIED!

		Quantity	Total
Haircutting Basics book (paperback)	@ **$16.95**	_____	_____
Haircutting Basics book (hardback)	@ **$24.95**	_____	_____
Haircutting Basics videotape	@ **$39.95**	_____	_____
Corte de Pelo Tecnica Basica (Spanish video)	@ **$39.95**	_____	_____
Paperback and videotape at package price	@ **$49.95**	_____	_____
Hardback and videotape at package price	@ **$56.95**	_____	_____

Sub-Total _____

Shipping: $1.00 for the first item and $0.50 for each additional item. _____

For videos, please circle. VHS   Beta   No COD orders please   **Total** _____

Name _____   Phone ( )_____

Address _____

City/State/Zip _____

_____ My check/money order is enclosed   _____ Bill my **American Express**   Card

Acct. # [ ][ ][ ][ ][ ][ ][ ][ ][ ][ ][ ][ ][ ][ ]   Expires _____   Signature _____

Mail to: Good Life Products, Inc., P. O. Box 5122, Hialeah, FL 33014-1122

Your are important to us. To help us make quality products for you by improving our future editions, tell us what you think.

Circle one: Are you an amateur, a cosmetology student, a graduate of cosmetology, a teacher or a salon owner?

Where did you see or buy this book?

Which haircuts did you practice?

Could you follow the steps easily?

Circle one: You found this book (very, little or average) informative.

How helpful were the drawings?

Did you find the technique easy enough to learn through a book?

What would you like to see or change in this book?

What other titles interest you?

Thank you for your cooperation.

Sincerely,

Diana Johnstone
Director